# HOW TO COPE
# SUCCESSFULLY WITH THE

# DIVERTICULITIS DIET

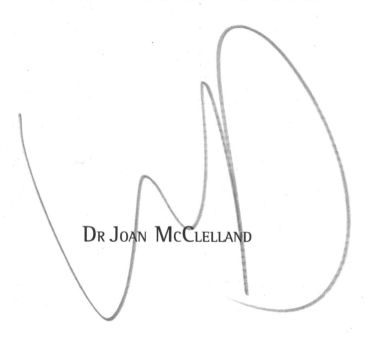

## Dr Joan McClelland

Wellhouse Publishing Ltd

First published in Great Britain in 2008 by
Wellhouse Publishing Ltd
31 Middle Bourne Lane
Lower Bourne
Farnham, Surrey GU10 3NH

## DISCLAIMER

The aim of this book is to provide general information only and should not
be treated as a substitute for the medical advice of your doctor or any other
health care professional. The publisher and author is not responsible or
liable for any diagnosis made by a reader based on the contents of this
book. Always consult your doctor if you are in any way concerned about
your health.

A catalogue record for this book is available from the British Library

ISBN: 978-1-903784-21-1

Also by Joan McClelland in the successfully series:
  *Diverticulitis*
  *Menopause*

Printed and bound in Great Britain by Creative Print & Design, Abertillery,
Wales NP13 3JW.

# Contents

# About the author:

Dr Joan McClelland studied medicine in Glasgow, Birmingham and London. For several years she worked with her husband in General Practice before specialising in psychiatry. She was elected a Fellow of the Royal College of Psychiatrists in 1982 and obtained diplomas in the history and philosophy of medicine in 1996 and 1998 respectively. Her particular interest is the interface between physical and psychological illness. Joan is now a full time author and lives near Churt, Surrey.

# Introduction

If you are a Westerner that is, you live in North America, Western Europe, Australia or New Zealand – and you are aged 50 or more, you are in the high-risk group for diverticular disorder. You had a 30 per cent likelihood at age 45, 40 per cent at 50 and 50 per cent plus when you hit 70. There are smaller areas of Western-type lifestyle, the likely sort for diverticulitis, among Jewish people all over the world, in modern Japan, and other sophisticated Asian countries like Singapore. It is a matter of soft living and a soft diet.

The behaviour that leads to diverticular disorder is lack of exercise involving the abdominal muscles that normally keep your figure in trim, and the automatic muscles of the colon, the lower part of the digestive passage itself. Without stimulus this becomes slack and baggy, with little pockets of food waste, the diverticula, bulging out from it. A minimum of three of these qualifies for a diagnosis of diverticulosis. Infection in one or more little pouches is called diverticulitis.

Diverticulosis and diverticulitis are the two forms of diverticular disorder. The former does not cause anything worse than discomfort, but diverticulitis is sharply painful and is often called left-sided appendicitis. The appendix is a blind alley, in fact a special diverticulum on the right side of the abdomen, and it is prone to stagnation of its contents and the development of infection. Adolescents and young adults are particularly susceptible to appendicitis, while the middle-aged and elderly more often get diverticulosis that develops into diverticulitis.

For a detailed description and explanation of diverticular disease, see my book *How to Cope Successfully with Diverticulitis*, Wellhouse Publishing, Farnham, UK, 2001.

The habits that make you vulnerable to diverticular disorder also lead to hiatus hernia at an age when the muscles of the digestive system are, like others, all becoming weaker and constipation is often beginning to be a problem. Increasing efforts are required to pass a motion.

Constipation, the sluggish movement of food waste along the intestine, is frequently the first indication of diverticular disease and may be accompanied by hiatus hernia. It is enhanced by:

- faulty diet: too little fibre; too much fattening food with too little bulk, e.g. chocolate
- dehydration, from inadequate fluid intake (common in older people)

- rushed modern lifestyle with insufficient patience to give the gut time to act
- reduced mobility, often because of arthritis: ordinary muscular exercise stimulates the intestines
- frequent travel, as in commuting, which may make it difficult to get to the loo
- some medicines, for instance pain-killers, antidepressants or iron pills
- illnesses such as hypothyroidism or diabetes
- sex: women are affected three times as often as men, i.e. less muscle work
- increasing age with weaker muscles.

The snags of modern living that underlie the current epidemic of obesity also impede the activity of the colon:

- being a couch potato – watching television
- being a mouse potato – the only exercise is clicking with the right index finger!
- supermarket shopping – everything under one roof
- ready-made meals – extra sweet and palatable
- less smoking – reduces appetite (but not to be recommended!)
- cars – even for the shortest journey
- labour-saving tools – washing machines, vacuum cleaners etc.

Symptoms of constipation are:

- bloating, discomfort
- backache, headache
- nausea
- passing a motion fewer than three times a week
- straining to pass a motion on at least 25 per cent of occasions
- haemorrhoids.

### How to Avoid Diverticular Disorder, Especially Diverticulitis, or to Lessen its Effects

There are two main ploys: exercise and, most importantly, diet.

### Exercise
This is simple, consisting of practising the use of the muscles of the abdomen, both internal and external. The external muscles are those that surround and support the abdomen, rather like a corset. They are

exercised by alternately drawing them in, holding for a count of ten, then relaxing them, and lying on your back and sitting up or raising your legs. Standing up with straight legs and touching your toes. Repeat each of these exercises ten times. *Ten times.* General bodily exercise also tones up these muscles; for instance, walking briskly for 30 minutes daily or 40 minutes three times a week.

Internal exercises use the muscles of the intestines themselves. You cannot tighten them voluntarily, but they can be stimulated by a diet that contains adequate amounts of fibre, giving them something solid to grip. This is the opposite of their slow, sluggish action in constipation. Fruit, especially citrus, and vegetables, especially the green, yellow and leafy types, provide a generous supply of fibre as well as vitamin C and antioxidants. Oats in particular and other wholegrain cereals are good sources of fibre.

Diet is the major key to beating diverticulitis and is the main subject of this book.

## General Dietary Requirements

General dietary requirements apply to everyone, whether or not you are focusing on diverticular problems. You need to have some of each of the three basic types of food:

- carbohydrates: fillers and the main suppliers of energy, they include bread, rice, cereals, pasta and potatoes
- proteins: necessary for growth and repair, these include foods derived from animal sources such as meat, fish, eggs and dairy produce, and vegetable products such as nuts and beans.
- fats: these provide concentrated nourishment, supplying more than twice as many calories as equivalent weights of protein or carbohydrate; they make other foods more palatable but easily lead to obesity
- fibre: this gives bulk to the diet.

Your daily intake of these various classes of food should be roughly divided as:

$1/3$ fruit and vegetables: 5 servings daily
$1/3$ bread, cereals, potatoes, pasta, rice: 6 servings daily
$1/6$ meat, fish, eggs and vegetable proteins such as beans
$1/6$ milk, dairy produce
$1/8$ fats and oils

7

Some foods and drinks provide calories but little else neither proteins, vitamins nor minerals. They are often supersweet, cooked in excess fats and oils, and in the case of drinks, often fizzy or with alcohol. They can be very palatable but should be eaten sparingly as they are valueless. In the case of fats, the saturated (animal) types should be avoided as far as possible.

Fibre provides no energy (fuel) but is valuable for its action in exercising the muscles of the gut. Since it passes through the body without being absorbed, it has little nutritional value.

Government advice on alcohol is 1 glass daily for women and 2 glasses for men, but a little wine in middle age may reduce the risk of heart disease.

Variety in the diet is necessary to ensure an adequate supply of *micronutrients*, substances necessary for health but required or only very small amounts: vitamins and minerals. Zinc and magnesium are among the latter.

Vitamins come in two types: water-soluble and fat-soluble. Vitamin C, ascorbic acid, is the commonest of the former, and is found in fruit and vegetables, while fat-soluble vitamin D enables the body to absorb calcium and maintain strong bones. This is the sunshine vitamin that we can manufacture in our skin with the help of ultra-violet light. There is a danger of running short of vitamin D with increasing age and lack of outdoor activity.

**Deficient Diet in the Apparently Rich, Industrialized Countries**
Between 4 and 25 per cent of the population in the European Union are living below the poverty line. Their babies are undersized at birth, and their older children shorter and less often breast-fed. As adults they tend to be overweight, with more lipids (fat) in their blood. They eat less lean meat, fruit and vegetables and wholemeal bread than the rest of us, and more fried foods, chips and sugary foods. This type of diet is likely to be deficient in:

- total energy, i.e. especially protein but with an excess of calories
- folates, found in liver, wheatgerm, soya, lettuce, eggs and cheese, vegetables
- vitamin C, the most important antioxidant, fighting wear-and -tear
- vitamin D, still a public health risk in Britain
- vitamin B12, cooperates with folate to make DNA
- iron, especially in women aged 15 to 50, affecting 33 per cent in Britain and causing definite anaemia in 11 per cent
- calcium, a lack of which causes osteoporosis, common in middle age onwards.

**Drugs that may cause malnutrition are:**

- aspirin and NSAIDs (non-steroidal anti-inflammatories) causing bleeding in the stomach and loss of iron
- digoxin, producing loss of appetite and could cause anorexia
- purgatives, leading to loss of half-digested food and potassium
- chemotherapy, which could cause anorexia
- diuretics (water tablets), possible loss of potassium
- slimming tablets, for instance amphetamines, increasing energy and cutting down appetite.

# The Glycaemic Index

The glycaemic index (GI) is a measure of the amount of sugar or its equivalent in your blood. The syllable *glyc* refers to the sugar, glucose, and *aem* means blood as in *haemorrhage*. Different foods have different glycaemic indices. Glucose is the standard with a glycaemic index of 100. The three main classes of nutrients, the macronutrients (*macro* = big) are proteins, carbohydrates and fats.

Proteins are used for building and repair work, while carbohydrates are the main fuel that produces the energy on which the body runs. They come in two main types: simple and complex. Simple carbohydrates are the sugars: for instance fructose in fruit, lactose in milk, sucrose, which is ordinary cane sugar, and glucose, the basic type. Sugars are rapidly absorbed into the bloodstream, giving an immediate boost to the blood sugar level and sometimes upsetting its control mechanism.

Complex carbohydrates include any except the sugars, for instance starches, and the carbohydrates in whole grains, fruits and vegetables. They are absorbed much more slowly than the simple type because they need digesting first.

A healthy diet with lashings of fruit and vegetables is beneficial to your body, especially the diverticular area of the bowels. This is because of their need for adequate supplies of fibre (see page 106) as a stimulus to functioning. Also, a wide variety of natural foods ensure that you get enough of vitamins B3, B6 and C in particular and also such minerals as zinc, iron and magnesium. Only tiny amounts are needed, but these are vital to your survival. The most valuable foods in this respect are nuts, seeds, oily fish like sardines, dark green vegetables, onions, peas and beans, asparagus and the brassica family. Oat bran is useful because of the soluble fibre it contains. This is the type that is important for checking the level of cholesterol in the blood, to the benefit of the whole body, but notably the heart and arteries. Unchecked, the harmful variety of cholesterol, LDL, builds up, blocking the blood vessels; it also leads to the modern plague of obesity.

Satiety, a feeling of fullness, is brought on by potatoes, boiled rather than chipped, but the fats from animal sources, for instance in dairy products and some meat dishes, stimulate the appetite despite their high nutritive value, more than twice that of equal weights of protein or carbohydrate. The body is designed to require a high blood sugar in situations of stress –

the fight or flight syndrome – or under the influence of such stimulants as a caffeine (tea and coffee), tobacco and alcohol. Unwelcome results are fatigue, anxiety, irritability, poor concentration and insomnia. Too much of easily absorbed, sweet carbohydrates such as chocolate causes the hormone insulin to be poured into the bloodstream, and there is a dramatic drop in the blood-sugar level. This in turn causes a craving for a 'fix' of something sweet – usually a fast food, processed to include a lot of hidden sugar and fat.

This is when the glycaemic index is a useful guide. A high index warns of an unstable blood sugar and the danger of too high a level too often or for too long  regardless of the calorie count. A low glycaemic index scores below 55 and a high index is over 70. If you eat one of the latter you need to take some low GI food at the same time, to slow down the release of sugar. Fatty foods have a low GI, but they are not to be recommended because of their high content of saturated fat, dangerous to the heart and arteries. Low GI is helpful for people with a tendency towards diabetes, high blood pressure and overweight.

## Low GI foods

**Fruits**

| | |
|---|---|
| cherries | 22 |
| grapefruit | 25 |
| pears | 37 |
| apples | 38 |
| oranges | 42 |
| bananas | 54 |
| apricots and other dried fruit | 31 |

**Vegetables and salad**

| | |
|---|---|
| broccoli | 10 |
| cabbage | 10 |
| lettuce | 10 |
| mushrooms | 10 |
| raw carrots | 10 |
| red peppers | 10 |

**Legumes**

| | |
|---|---|
| soya beans | 14 |
| red split lentils | 18 |
| canned baked beans | 45 |
| green peas | 48 |

**Grains**

| | |
|---|---|
| pearl barley | 31 |
| rye | 34 |
| brown basmati rice | 52 |

**Bread**

| | |
|---|---|
| mixed grain | 48 |
| rye bread | 50 |

**Pasta**

| | |
|---|---|
| vermicelli etc. | 35 |

**Dairy products**

| | |
|---|---|
| skimmed or full-fat milk | 27 |
| low-fat yoghurt | 14 |
| low-fat fruit yoghurt | 33 |

**Sponge cake**          **46**

**Bran cereal**          **42**

## Moderate GI Foods

**Fruit**

| | |
|---|---|
| mangoes | 56 |
| fresh apricots | 57 |
| pineapple | 66 |

**Vegetables**

| | |
|---|---|
| sweetcorn | 55 |
| new potatoes | 57 |
| beetroot | 64 |
| mashed or boiled potatoes | 70 |

**Grains**

| | |
|---|---|
| white basmati rice | 58 |
| buckwheat | 55 |

**Bread**

| | |
|---|---|
| white pitta bread | 58 |
| hamburger bun | 61 |
| wholemeal bread | 69 |

**Pasta**

durum wheat          55

**Bakery**

pastry               59
croissant            67
crumpet              69

**Breakfast cereals**

muesli               56
porridge             61
All Bran             30
Shredded Wheat       75
Weetabix             69
Biscuits             55-64

**Sugary foods**

extra fruity jam     55
honey                58
table sugar          64

**Soft drinks**

still orange         66
fizzy orange         68
Ice cream            61

## High GI Foods – Watch Out!

**Fruit**

melon                72
dates                99

**Vegetables**

swedes               72
chips                75
baked potatoes       85
cooked carrots       85
parsnips             97

**Grains**

polished rice        88

## Bread
| | |
|---|---|
| white bagel | 72 |
| white loaf | 78 |
| baguette | 95 |

## Bakery
| | |
|---|---|
| doughnuts | 76 |
| waffles | 76 |

## Breakfast cereals
| | |
|---|---|
| Wheat Bran Flakes plus dried fruit | 71 |
| Puffed Wheat | 74 |
| Rice Crispies | 82 |
| Corn Flakes | 83 |
| High glucose sports drinks | 95 (pure glucose rates 100) |

## Legumes
| | |
|---|---|
| broad beans | 79 |

## Low GI Recipes

### Nutty Cereal
115 g/ 4 oz flaked almonds
115 g/ 4 oz chopped hazelnuts
115 g/ 4 oz jumbo oats
115 g/ 4 oz chopped dried apricots
85 g/ 3 oz sunflower seeds

Toast the nuts on a baking sheet, cool, then mix all the ingredients together. They will keep for a few days in an airtight container.

Serve with sliced banana and strawberries, raspberries in season, or sliced apple. Contains omega-6 oils.

### Eggs Florentine (rather a fandangle to do, but a very classy, healthy dish)
450 g/ 1 lb spinach, washed and shaken
55 g/ 2 oz butter or olive oil spread
55 g/ 2 oz sliced button mushrooms
55 g/ 2 oz toasted pine kernels
1 spring onion, chopped
2 eggs

25 g/ 1 oz wholemeal flour
300 ml/ 10 fl oz milk
85 g/ 3 oz grated cheddar cheese

Heat the washed spinach without water for 2-3 minutes, then chop. Cook the mushrooms for 2 minutes in half the butter, then add the pine kernels and spring onion and cook for a further 2 minutes. Scatter over the spinach. Meanwhile poach the eggs and put on top of the spinach. Melt the remaining butter and stir in the flour. Gradually stir in the milk, add half the cheese and heat until the mixture thickens. Pour over the eggs, sprinkle with the remaining cheese and cook in the oven for 20 minutes or until golden brown and bubbling.

   Spinach is rich in folic acid, a B vitamin needed for healing and growth, especially in pregnancy.

## Moroccan Lamb
450 g/ 1 lb lean leg of lamb, cut into 1-inch cubes
1½ tsp black pepper
15 ml/ 1 tbsp olive oil
1 large onion, peeled and diced
1-2 cloves of garlic, crushed (optional)
2 tomatoes, skinned and, sliced
1 tbsp hot pepper paste
425 ml/ ¾ pt water
400 g/ 15 oz can of chickpeas
350 g/ 12 oz peeled pumpkin, cut into 1-inch cubes
1 tbsp chopped mint
1 tbsp chopped coriander
squeeze of lemon if available

Cover the lamb with pepper and brown in the oil, add the onion and garlic and cook in a non-stick pan until the onion is soft and slightly brown, then add tomatoes, hot pepper paste and water. Bring to a simmer, then cover and cook for 1½ hours. Add chickpeas and pumpkin and cook for another 15 minutes. Then add the mint, coriander and lemon – and, hey presto, the most delicious lamb you've ever tasted! Serve with flatbread.

## Compote of Plums in Rosemary Syrup
150 ml/ ¼ pt red wine
50 g/ 2 oz caster sugar
sprig of rosemary
bay leaf

1 strip each of lemon and orange rind
2 cloves
5 cm/2-inch cinnamon stick
500 g/18 oz stoned red plums

Put all the ingredients except the plums into a pan and bring to the boil. Simmer until the sugar has dissolved, then add the plums, cover and cook gently until plums are tender. Remove the plums and serve warm or cold with low-fat yoghurt.

## Medium GI recipes

### Vegetable Biryani
2 tbsp vegetable oil
3 cloves
3 cracked cardamom pods
1 chopped onion
2 crushed garlic cloves (optional)
2 fresh red chillies, de-seeded and chopped
1-inch chunk of root ginger, grated
115 g/4 oz cauliflower florets
175 g/6 oz broccoli florets
115 g/4oz chopped French beans
1 tbsp chopped coriander
400 g/14 oz canned chopped tomatoes
150 ml/5 fl oz vegetable stock
115 g/4 oz okra (lady's fingers)
115 g/4 oz brown basmati rice

Heat the oil gently in a pan with spices, onion, carrots, garlic, chillies and ginger. Stir for 5 minutes. Add all the vegetables except the okra. Stir and cook for 5 minutes, then add tomatoes and stock and cook for a further 10 minutes. Add the okra and cook for 8-10 minutes more, then stir in the coriander and drain off excess liquid.

Layer the vegetables and cooked rice and press down in a deep dish. Leave for 5 minutes then tip into a warmed serving dish.

Cauliflower is reputed to be a good source of vitamin B6, and to benefit both mental health and mood.

### Crème Brûlé
250 g/9 oz mascarpone cheese
200 ml/7 oz crème fraîche

300 g/ 10 oz mixed soft fruits as available
      (raspberries, cherries, strawberries)
2 tbsp dark muscovado sugar

Cream the cheese until soft, then gradually stir in the crème fraîche. Spoon the mixture over the fruit, covering it completely. Chill in the fridge. Sprinkle with sugar, then heat under the grill until caramelized. Serve at once or chill first.

### Duck Salad with Mango Salsa
2 duck breast fillets
200 g/ 7 oz assorted salad leaves
110 g/ 4 oz mange-tout, shredded or fine green beans, cooked
For the salsa:
1 mango, diced
small bunch of mint, chopped
small bunch of coriander, chopped
juice of 1 lime
1 red onion, diced
1 chilli, de-seeded and finely chopped
3 tomatoes, diced
freshly ground black pepper to taste
pinch of salt

Preheat the oven to 190C°/375°F/gas mark 5. Score criss-crosses close together on the skin of the duck to release the fat when cooking. Put the duck, skin side down, in an ovenproof frying pan over a medium heat and cook for 4-5 minutes. Turn the duck over and cook for 1-2 minutes. Transfer to the oven and cook for a further 5-10 minutes, depending on how well-done you like it (when the duck is slightly undercooked it will feel springy to the touch and the flesh will be pinkish, but if it is fully cooked it will be firm and less pink). Meanwhile, combine the ingredients for the salsa and season to taste. Remove from the oven and leave for 5-10 minutes before slicing. Finally, arrange the slices of duck on a bed of salad leaves and mange-tout. Serve with the salsa. (Serves 4 )

### Dolcelatte and Vegetable Cheesecake
For the base:
55 g/ 2 oz ground almonds
55 g/ 2 oz fresh wholemeal breadcrumbs
55 g/ 2 oz finely chopped toasted hazelnuts
55 g/ 2 oz freshly grated Parmesan cheese

55 g / 2 oz unsalted melted butter
For the filling:
10 g / $\frac{1}{4}$ oz sun-dried tomatoes
115 g / 4 oz baby asparagus spears
115 g / 4 oz broccoli
1 red pepper, skinned, de-seeded and cut into thin strips
140 g / 5 oz dolcelatte cheese
450 g / 1 lb mascarpone cheese
3 eggs

Preheat the oven to 180°C/350°F/gas mark 4. Mix the almonds, breadcrumbs, hazelnuts and Parmesan cheese together in a bowl. Stir the melted butter into the nut mixture, mix well, then press into the base of an 8-inch (20 cm) tin. Bake for 15 minutes, then remove from the oven and reserve meanwhile put the tomatoes into an ovenproof bowl, cover with almost boiling water, leave for 20 minutes, then drain and chop. Trim the asparagus and, if thick, cut in half. Cut the broccoli into long, thin spears, including the stalk. Cook both together in very lightly salted boiling water for 3 minutes, then drain, plunge into cold water and leave to cool. Drain again. Arrange the vegetables and red pepper over the nut base and crumble over half the dolcelatte cheese. Cream the mascarpone cheese in a bowl until soft, then gradually beat in the eggs. When smooth, pour over the vegetables and crumble the remaining dolcelatte cheese over the top. Put the tin on a baking tray and bake until set, approximately 35-40 minutes. Remove from the oven and, when cool, remove the cheesecake from the tin – a fiddly business, but the end result is worthwhile.

Using ground nuts instead of grain for the base reduces the amount of carbohydrate and slows down the release of sugars into the bloodstream. This makes for a low GI but a high calorie count, with 65 g fat of which 8 g is saturated.

## BLT Sandwich
4 slices of granary bread
Butter or low-fat spread
1 tbsp mayonnaise
lettuce
2 tomatoes, sliced
4 rashers of streaky bacon, well grilled
75 g / 3 oz Somerset Brie, sliced, or Stilton, Cheshire, Cheddar or
    Leicester

Spread 2 slices of bread with butter and 2 slices with mayonnaise. Arrange lettuce, tomato, bacon and cheese on top. Cover with remaining bread. Makes an ideal packed lunch: medium GI, medium fat, no cooking. Serves 2.

An excellent book that explains the glycaemic index and gives you tasty, healthy recipes is *Antony Worrall Thompson's GI Diet,* with Dr Mabel Blades and Jane Suthering, published by Kyle Cathie Ltd.

# Vegetables

Vegetables are the most important foodstuffs for those suffering from diverticular problems or aiming to avoid them. The fibre in vegetables provides the stimulus to keep the colon working steadily and healthily, and especially in the elderly it keeps constipation at bay. The word vegetable , appropriately, comes from the Latin *vegere*, to be active. Vigil and vigour come from the same root. Types of soluble fibre contained in vegetables are pectin, guar and oat fibre and these produce moderate reductions in blood cholesterol: 5 g per day of these fibres causes a reduction of about 5 per cent. Vegetables and fruit contain around 1 per cent pectin, which means that four portions provide 5 g. Oatmeal, oat bran and legumes all contain soluble fibre. Vegetables at a main meal should cover about three-quarters of the plate.

Most vegetable foods are low in protein, except for soya. Using vegetable instead of animal protein usually reduces the blood cholesterol level, particularly the more dangerous LDL type. One snag in eating vegetables is that they taste better with salt, and there is a temptation not only to cook them with salt but to sprinkle it generously on the food in front of you. Apart from cakes and desserts there is hardly a recipe in the cook book that does not include salt. Processing food usually increases the salt content. Salt is chemically sodium chloride, NaCl, so in the chart below the numbers refer to amounts of salt.

|             | Fresh | Canned | Frozen |
|-------------|-------|--------|--------|
| Peas        | 5 mg  | 394 mg | 147 mg |
| Green beans | 4 mg  | 361 mg | 19 mg  |

The passage of time and exposure to the air have a disastrous effect on the vitamin content of various vegetables. Lettuce loses 50 per cent of its vitamin C a week after it is picked, other vegetables similarly. The moral is to eat fresh vegetables just as soon as possible after they are picked. Cooking destroys vitamins, especially Vitamin C, ascorbic acid.

The Queen of British cookery, Mrs Isabella Beeton, recognised the value of vegetables in 1861, in her famous book *Home Cooking*. She wrote:

Persons in the flower of youth, having healthy stomachs and leading active lives [note, even in Mrs Beeton s day] may eat all sorts of vegetables without inconvenience, save, of course, in excess. The digestive functions possess great energy during the period of youth, and the body, to develop itself, needs nourishment. Physical exercise gives an appetite which it is necessary to satisfy and vegetables cannot resist the vigorous action of the gastric organs. But for aged persons, the sedentary or the delicate, it is quite otherwise. Then the gastric power has considerably diminished, the digestive organs have lost their energy, the process of digestion is consequently slower and the least excess at table is followed by derangement of the stomach for several days. Those who generally digest vegetables with difficulty should eat them reduced to a pulp or puree, that is to say, with their skins and tough fibres removed.

Subjected to this process, vegetables which, when entire, would create flatulence and wind are then comparatively harmless.

## Vegetable Recipes

### Mrs Beeton's Asparagus Pudding
150 g/ 6 oz asparagus tips
25 g/ 1 oz ham
4 eggs
30 ml/ 2 tbsp flour
salt and pepper to taste
25 g/ 1 oz soft buttermilk

Cut the asparagus into pea-sized pieces and mince the ham finely with asparagus. Beat together the eggs and flour, adding salt and pepper to taste, then add the asparagus and ham. Add buttermilk until the batter has a thick consistency. Pour the mixture into a greased 1-pt basin. Cover with a double layer of buttered greaseproof paper or foil. Steam gently for 2 hours. Serves 3 or 4.

### Roast Asparagus
While Mrs Beeton's pudding is quite complicated to cook, Roast Asparagus is a doddle but a little more special than just serving the shoots with melted butter.
2 or 3 bunches of asparagus
butter
olive oil
pepper and salt
2 tbsp white sugar
1 lemon

Trim the tough white part of the stalks from the asparagus. Place the spears flat in a baking dish, dot with butter, splash with olive oil, sprinkle with salt and freshly-ground pepper and the sugar. Put the dish in a hot oven, then reduce to medium heat for 20 minutes, uncovered, or until the asparagus begins to get crisp. Remove the cooked asparagus with a fish slice and squeeze the juice of the lemon over them. Top with flakes of Parmesan and serve.

Asparagus is from the Greek asparagus, but from the mid-17th century until the 20th century it was called sparrow-grass . It has a short season in May and June and should not be missed.

### Aubergines with Yoghurt
2 aubergines
2 crushed cloves of garlic
60 ml/ 4 tbsp olive oil
250 g/ 10 oz low-fat natural yoghurt

Cut the unpeeled aubergines in $\frac{1}{4}$-inch slices, sprinkle with salt and leave for 30 minutes, then fry until soft. Stir the crushed garlic into the yoghurt and pour over the aubergines. Serve hot.

'Aubergine' comes from the Sanskrit *vatinganah* meaning 'wind-go', a reference to the flatulent effect of many vegetables. Americans call it the 'eggplant'.

### Stuffed Tomatoes Provencal
8 tomatoes
50 g/ 2 oz onions
clove of garlic (optional)
25 g/ 1 oz butter or vegetable oil
30 ml/ 2 tbsp olive oil
75100 g/ 3 oz soft white breadcrumbs
30 ml/ 2 tbsp chopped parsley
Seasoning to taste

Halve the tomatoes, remove seeds and juice, and place in an ovenproof dish. Skin and chop the onion and crush the garlic, then fry in butter. Add the breadcrumbs and parsley, season and pour over the tomatoes then drizzle the tomatoes with the olive oil. Heat in the oven 190°C/375°F/gas mark 5 for 20-25 minutes or until the crumbs are lightly browned.

**Brussels Sprouts with Peppers and Potatoes**
15 ml/ 1 tbsp vegetable oil
1 onion, chopped
large potato, cubed
bay leaf
450 g/ 1 lb brussels sprouts
1 red pepper, cut in 1 cm/ ½-inch pieces
60 ml/ 2 fl oz vegetable stock
freshly ground pepper
30 ml/ 2 tbsp chopped fresh parsley

Warm the vegetable oil over a medium heat and fry the onion, potato and bay leaf for 2-3 minutes. Add the brussels sprouts, red pepper and stock. Cover and cook until the sprouts and potatoes are tender. Season with pepper to taste. Serve sprinkled with parsley.

Brussels sprouts – *choux de Bruxelles* – have been connected with the town since 1223 and are the traditional accompaniment to Christmas turkey or chicken.

**Colcannon**
450 g/ 1 lb shredded cabbage
450 g / 1 lb potatoes, halved
2 leeks, chopped
150 ml/¼ pt milk
pepper and salt
pinch of ground mace
25 g/ 1 oz butter

Boil the cabbage in water, drain and keep warm. Meanwhile put the potatoes and leeks into a pan with the milk. Bring to the boil, cover and simmer until soft. Mash the potatoes and leeks, season, and mix in the cabbage. Reheat. Serve in a dish with melted butter.

The word 'cabbage' comes from the Old French *caboche*, meaning head. Kohlrabi is a kind of cabbage with a turnip-shaped stem, introduced from Germany in the early 19th century; its name means literally 'cabbage turnip'.

**Mange-tout**
This is the French for 'eat-all', but the French themselves call this type of pea *pois gourmand* and give you French beans if you ask for mange-tout! Mange-tout to us consists of nearly flat pods with tiny immature peas still

inside; the Americans call them 'snow peas', and we used to call them 'sugar snaps' or 'sugar peas'. They need topping and stringing and are cooked like ordinary peas. They are delicious with any main meal and full of vitamins and plant protein.

## Spinach Soup
450 g/ 1lb spinach
25 g/ 1 oz cornflour
50 g / 2 oz butter
pinch of salt, pepper and nutmeg
150 ml/¹⁄₄ pt full-cream milk
croutons

Wash and cook the spinach without added water until tender. Sieve or liquidize. Cook the cornflour for 1 minute in the melted butter, then add the spinach puře. Season with salt, pepper and nutmeg. Stir in the warmed milk. Serve with croutons of fried bread.

Spinach is steeped in history, from 6th-century Persia as *aspanakh* and in China as *poh t'sai* (Persian vegetable). As well as vitamin C, spinach is rich in iron: the darker the colour the better.

## Turnip and Apple Purée
1 small turnip (about 550 g/1¹⁄₄ lb)
1 large apple, peeled, cored and cut into chunks
60 g/2 ¹⁄₄ oz low-fat natural yoghurt
15 ml/ 1 tsp unsaturated vegetable fat
pinch of salt, pepper and nutmeg

Steam the turnip until tender (about 20 minutes). Add the apple and cook for a further 5-10 minutes. Drain. Purée in a liquidizer and add the yoghurt, fat and seasoning. Reheat.

The Latin *napus* refers to the 'nip' of turnip or parsnip, but no one knows where 'tur' or 'par' come from!

## Mushroom-Stuffed Courgettes
2 medium-sized courgettes
10 ml/ 2 tsp unsaturated margarine
75 g/ 3 oz mushrooms, finely chopped
15 ml/ 1 tbsp onion or shallots, finely chopped
fresh parsley, finely chopped
freshly ground pepper and pinch of salt
grated Parmesan cheese

Cut courgettes into 2.5 cm (1-inch) lengths and steam for 5 minutes or until tender-crisp. Scoop out a small hollow from each piece of courgette and set aside. Melt the margarine and cook the mushrooms and onions or shallots in a non-stick pan until tender. Stir in the parsley and seasoning. Arrange the courgette pieces in an ovenproof dish and spoon the mushroom filling into the hollows of the courgettes. Cover with foil and bake at 180°C/ 350°F/gas mark 4 for 15-20 minutes. Serve in a dish sprinkled with Parmesan.

'Courgette' comes from the French word *courge* and the Italian *zucca*; both mean 'gourd'.

### Lettuce and Herb Sauce
6 small lettuces
25 g/ 1 oz butter or vegetable spread
25 g/ 1 oz flour
250 ml/½ pt stock
10 ml/ 2 tsp chopped chives
10 ml/ 2 tsp chopped parsley
bay leaf

Trim and wash the lettuces, then plunge into boiling water for 2 minutes. Drain, then refresh in cold water. Melt the butter in a saucepan and stir in the flour for 1 minute; avoid browning. Stir in stock, chives and parsley and the bay leaf. Bring to the boil and heat gently for about 30 minutes or until it thickens. Remove the bay leaf before serving.

### Carrot and Cheese Bake
50 g/ 2 oz butter or spread
75 g/ 3 oz porridge oats
150 g/ 5 oz English cheddar cheese, grated
400 g/ 14 oz carrots, grated
25 g/ 1 oz wholemeal flour
45 ml/ 3 tbsp milk
1.25 ml/ ¼ tsp dried thyme
15 ml/ 1 tbsp sesame seeds
15 ml/ 1 tbsp poppy seeds

Mix all the ingredients together except for the sesame seeds and poppy seeds. Spoon into a greased ovenproof dish, pressing well in. Sprinkle the sesame and poppy seeds over the top and bake for 30 minutes.

## Vegetarian Dishes

These recipes all include vegetable protein, partly replacing animal derivatives: milk, meat, fish, cheese and eggs. The likeliest deficiency is iron.

### Vegetable and Nut Cobbler

150 g/ 5 oz butter
175 g/ 6 oz cauliflower florets
6 baby onions
175 g/ 6 oz carrots, sliced
1 medium parsnip, sliced
175 g/ 6 oz green beans, sliced
400 g/ 14 oz can of butter beans, drained
1 vegetable stock cube
568 ml/ 1 pt milk
240 g/ $8\frac{1}{2}$ oz wholemeal self-raising flour
100 g/ 4 oz Red Leicester cheese, grated
freshly ground pepper
10 ml/ 2 tsp baking powder
50 g/ 2 oz chopped walnuts

Cover and cook raw vegetables in 1 oz butter for 10 minutes. Add the butter beans, stock cube, 459 ml/$\frac{3}{4}$pt milk, 15 g/ $\frac{1}{2}$oz flour, half the cheese and seasoning. Transfer to an ovenproof dish, cover and bake for 15 minutes 220°C/425°F/gas mark 7. To make the scone topping, sift the remaining flour and baking powder and rub in the remaining butter to look like breadcrumbs, then add the nuts. Stir in the remaining milk to make a soft dough. Chill for 10 minutes. Roll out on a floured board to 1 cm/$\frac{1}{2}$ inch thick and cut into 12 rounds or squares. Take the dish from oven, remove the cover and place the scones on top. Sprinkle with remaining cheese and return to oven for 15 minutes at 180°C/350°F/gas mark 4 or until the scones are golden brown. This is a luxury dish!

### Gloucester Pie

8 slices of brown bread, buttered and with crusts removed
100 g/ 4 oz thinly sliced Double Gloucester cheese
225 g/ 8 oz sliced tomatoes
150 ml/$\frac{1}{4}$pt milk
1 egg
5 ml/ 1 tsp made mustard
freshly ground pepper
green salad

Sandwich the bread with cheese and tomatoes. Cut each sandwich into 4 triangles and arrange in an ovenproof dish. Beat together the milk, egg, mustard and season to taste, pour over the sandwiches. Allow to stand for 30 minutes or until the bread absorbs all the liquid, then bake in a pre-heated oven 190°C/375°F/gas mark 5 for 25-30 minutes or until the top is crisp and golden. Serve with a green salad. Serves 4.

## Peanut Mince

1 large onion, chopped
100 g/ 4 oz mushrooms, chopped
1 celery stick, sliced
1 large carrot, grated
25 g/ 1 oz butter or vegetable oil spread
2.5 ml/ ½ tsp yeast extract
225 g/ 8 oz coarsely chopped peanuts
150 ml/ ¼ pt milk
150 ml/ ¼ pt vegetable stock or water
75 g/ 3 oz rolled oats
freshly ground pepper
30 ml/ 2 tbsp chopped parsley

Fry the vegetables in butter until pale gold. Stir in the yeast extract, peanuts, milk and stock or water. Bring to the boil, cover and simmer until the vegetables are tender, then add the oats and simmer for 4-5 minutes uncovered, until the mixture is thick. Season to taste and stir in the chopped parsley. Serve with mashed potato and green vegetables.

The mixture in this recipe substitutes for meat.

## Jacket Potato

4 large potatoes, about 175 g/ 6 oz each
50 g/ 2 oz butter (or sour cream and chives)

Wash, scrub and dry the potatoes. Prick well all over, or make several slits in each one. Microwave for 10-13 minutes (depending on manufacturers guidelines), turning half way, or bake in an ordinary pre-heated oven at 180°C/350°F/gas mark 4 for 1 ¼ hours or until they feel tender to pressure. Cut a large cross in each potato and put a piece of butter in each one. Serve immediately. Serves 4.

Optional fillings: cheddar cheese (vegetarian), baked beans, sardines, tuna with or without mayonnaise. Any but the last two alternatives are suitable for vegetarians.

Roast Butternut Squash
1 large squash
zest of an orange
pinch of cinnamon

Cut into halves and de-seed. Place on a non-stick baking tray skin-side down, sprinkled with orange zest and cinnamon, and bake in a pre-heated oven at 220°C/425°F/gas mark 7 for 40 minutes or until tender. Delicious as a side vegetable.

## Mushroom Risotto
3 tbsp olive oil
1 onion, peeled and finely chopped
1 punnet of mushrooms, sliced
1 clove of garlic, peeled and chopped
450 g/1 lb risotto rice
1.7 l/3 pt hot vegetable stock
1 tbsp fresh thyme sprigs
6 spring onions, chopped
minimal seasoning
fresh Parmesan shavings

Gently heat 2 tbsp of the oil in a saucepan. Cook the finely chopped onion until softened but not browned. Add about three-quarters of the mushrooms plus the garlic and cook for 2 minutes. Stir in the rice and go on cooking until the grains are translucent and glossy. Turn the heat down and add the stock, one tablespoon at a time. All the liquid must be absorbed gradually. Stir continuously for 20-25 minutes. Add half the thyme with the last spoonful of stock. Season slightly, cover and leave to stand. Put the remaining oil into a small pan, add the remaining mushrooms and the spring onions. Cover them with oil but do not cook. Add these to the rest of the risotto. Serve, sprinkled with the last of the thyme and shavings of Parmesan.

## Steamed Fresh Vegetables
For this you could use a mixture of leftover vegetables – for instance, half a stalk of broccoli or cauliflower, a few odd mushrooms and a couple of carrots and parsnips. Substitutes or additions include celery, fennel, red or green pepper, mange-tout, brussels sprouts, courgettes or cabbage.

2 medium carrots, peeled and sliced
2 medium parsnips, peeled and sliced

1 stalk of broccoli in florets
8 mushrooms
1 tbsp unsaturated spread
freshly ground pepper, touch of salt

Steam the carrots and parsnips for 3-5 minutes until tender or al dente. Add the broccoli and mushrooms and steam for 3 minutes or until the broccoli is bright green. Transfer to a serving dish and add the spread. Season and toss to mix.

This is a good supplier of niacin, excellent for fibre and vitamins A and C.

## Roast Parsnips
2 parsnips
4 carrots
1 tbsp unsaturated spread
freshly ground pepper and pinch of salt
pinch of cumin (optional)
1 tbsp water

Peel the parsnips and carrots, cut in half crossways, then lengthways in strips. Put in a baking dish and dot with spread. Season to taste. Add water, cover and bake for an hour or until the vegetables are tender. Serves 4.

Parsnips form their roots in November and, as the weather gets colder, they store energy in the form of sugar and therefore taste sweet. Roast parsnips and honey are a favourite country recipe.

## Leek Bake
55 g/ 2 oz unsalted butter, melted
115 g/ 4 oz ground almonds
55 g/ 2 oz toasted, chopped hazelnuts
25 g/ 1 oz sesame seeds
85 g/ 3 oz mature Cheddar cheese, grated
1 tbsp virgin olive oil
350 g/ 12 oz leeks, thinly sliced
1 large red pepper, skinned, de-seeded and cut into strips
1 orange pepper, skinned, de-seeded and cut into strips
85 g/ 3 oz button mushrooms, sliced
250 g/ 9 oz low-fat crème fraîche
1 tbsp chopped fresh oregano
seasoning

Pre-heat oven to 160°C/325°F/gas mark 3. Mix together the butter, nuts, sesame seeds and half the cheese in a bowl. Press the mixture into the bottom of a 1½ pt ovenproof gratin dish. Bake for 15 minutes or until the top is golden. Meanwhile, heat the oil in a big frying pan, add the crème fraîche, leeks, peppers and mushrooms and cook for 5 minutes, stirring a few times. Stir in the oregano, salt and pepper to taste. Remove the nut base from the oven. Spread the crème fraîche over the nut base and sprinkle with the rest of the cheese. Bake in the oven for 15-20 minutes or until the cheese is golden-brown and bubbling.

Oregano is a natural antiseptic and it calms the gut, especially after a heavy meal. It belongs to the mint family. This dish has a low glycaemic index.

**Baked Big Mushrooms**
4 large field mushrooms
200 g/ 7 oz canned red kidney beans, drained and rinsed
4 spring onions
1 fresh red jalapeno chilli, de-seeded and finely chopped
1 tbsp finely grated lemon rind
1 tbsp fresh parsley and extra sprigs to garnish
seasoning
85 g/ 3 oz coarsely grated courgettes
85 g/ 3 oz coarsely grated carrots
55 g/ 2 oz pine kernels, toasted
40 g/ 1½ oz raisins
300 ml/ 10 fl oz vegetable stock
For the sauce:
150 ml/ 5 fl oz Greek-style yoghurt
1 tbsp fresh parsley, chopped
1 tbsp grated lemon rind
seasoning

Preheat the oven to 180°C/350°F/gas mark 4. Peel the mushrooms, remove the stalks, trim and rinse them. Put the beans, mushroom stalks, spring onions, chilli, lemon rind, parsley, pepper to taste and a pinch of salt into a food processor and process for 2 minutes. Empty the mixture into a bowl and add the courgette, carrots, pine kernels and raisins. Mix well and stuff the mushroom cups generously. Arrange the stuffed mushrooms in an ovenproof dish, carefully pour round the stock and cover with foil. Bake for 30 minutes, removing the foil for the last 10 minutes. Meanwhile, to make the sauce, blend all the ingredients together in a small serving dish. Serve the mushrooms hot together with the sauce and garnished with parsley sprigs.

Mushrooms are high in protein and minerals, encourage the beneficial bacteria in the gut and boost the immune system. Meat substitutes are often based on mushrooms or other fungi.

## Kale Sautéed with Garlic
butter for frying
2 cloves of garlic, chopped
minced onion
chopped kale, handful
2 – 3 tbsp vegetable or chicken stock
juice of one lemon
seasoning

Melt the butter over medium heat, add the garlic and onion and sauté for 1 minute. Add the kale to the pan and sauté for 2 minutes, stirring constantly, until the kale is wilted. Add 2-3 tablespoons of stock and simmer until the kale is tender. Sprinkle with lemon juice and season to taste. Serve as a side dish to a main course.

Kale is a superstar for food values, abounding in vitamins A and C, iron and calcium. Use it like spinach or other green vegetables, but cook for a little longer to soften the tough outer leaves. It can be added to soup for the last 10 minutes of cooking time. Alternatively, simmer in a little stock and mix with white beans and bacon. Serve on toast, drizzled with olive oil.

## Egg Flower Soup with Broccoli or Pac Choi
750 ml/1½ pt chicken or vegetable stock, preferably fresh
2 handfuls of pac choi strips or broccoli florets
2 eggs, beaten
2 tsp soy sauce or tamari
1 tsp sesame oil
chilli oil or pepper to taste

Bring the stock to the boil and add the pac choi or broccoli. Cook for a few minutes until tender. Remove the vegetables to a dish. Return the stock to the boil and drizzle in the beaten eggs, stirring once to make 'egg flowers' – a magic creation. Remove from the heat, add the vegetables and let them stand for 2 minutes. Stir in the soy sauce, sesame oil and chilli or pepper to taste. Serve immediately.

## Best Choices in Fruit and Vegetables

Go for:

- fresh fruits and vegetables (top choice)
- frozen fruits and vegetables (second best)
- canned fruits and vegetables including pulses, e.g. sweetcorn, tomatoes, peas, baked beans, red kidney beans, chickpeas (next best, but still a good choice)
- unsweetened juices
- tomato purée
- fruits canned with natural juice

Avoid:

- avocados
- canned vegetables with high salt or sodium content
- sweetened juices
- canned fruits in heavy syrup

## Keeping Vitamins and Minerals in Fruit and Vegetables

Vitamins B and C and some minerals are soluble in water, so it is good sense to cook vegetables with a minimum of it. Don't soak them in cold water before cooking but plunge them into boiling water or steam them, so that as little as possible of the valuable vitamins and minerals is lost. Sugar is also water-soluble, so applying the same method of cooking allows the vegetables to keep more of their natural sweetness.

# Fruit

Fruit and vegetables share plentiful fibre. Wheat fibre, found in bran and wholemeal breads, has no effect on blood cholesterol, but soluble fibre, including pectin and guar, in fruits does help to lower blood cholesterol and is good for the heart and blood pressure. Fruits contain flavonoids and other antioxidants, vitamin C and folate, especially in raw, fresh fruit.

'Fresh' is something of a misnomer. Most of the fruit labelled 'fresh' in the shops and supermarkets comes from abroad or, if it has been grown locally, has been stored for weeks or months. Bananas are picked green in the tropics, then shipped and stored at an even 13°C, and finally ripened with ethylene gas. Oranges are picked ripe, shipped and stored at a lower 3°C in dry air with a raised carbon dioxide level. Their skins must be protected from mould infection, usually by treating them with fungicides mixed with waxes after they have been washed. Although they have been in artificial environments, these fruits are alive and their cells are absorbing oxygen and producing carbon dioxide. Sulphur dioxide is used as a preservative for dried fruits such as figs, prunes, apricots.

Health departments both in the United Kingdom and the United States recommend a high daily intake of fruit and vegetables: 5-6 portions a day, preferably a variety. One serving of fruit is a medium-sized peach, orange, apple or banana, or 2 plums, 3-4 strawberries or 5 cherries, or half or a quarter of a melon. Vegetables are healthy but fruit is nearly always a treat!

## Recipes

**Apple and Raspberry Crisp**
675 g/1½ lb apples, peeled and sliced
1 pkt (300 g/ 12 oz) frozen raspberries
60 g/2½ oz granulated sugar (or less if possible)
2 tbsp plain white flour
2 tsp cinnamon
For the topping:
75 g/ 3 oz quick-cooking rolled oats
40 g/1½ oz brown sugar
1 tsp cinnamon
50 g/ 2 oz saturated margarine

Combine the apples and raspberries, thawed or frozen, in a 3-pt baking dish. In a small bowl combine the sugar, flour and cinnamon. Add to the fruit and toss to mix. To make the topping, combine the rolled oats, sugar and cinnamon. With knives or a blender, cut in the margarine until crumbly. Sprinkle over the top of the fruit mixture. Bake at 180°C/350°F/ gas mark 4 for 55 minutes, or microwave on high for 15 minutes, until the mixture is bubbling and the fruit only just tender. Serve either warm or cold. Serves 8.

Alternative: for apple, pear and apricot crisp, use 450 g/ 1 lb peeled and sliced apples, 225 g/ 8 oz peeled and sliced pears and 50 g/ 2 oz coarsely chopped dried apricots.

This is a very low-fat recipe, excellent for fibre and good for vitamin C. Adding oatmeal increases the fibre and enhances the flavour.

## Pears, Blue Cheese and Avocado Salad
2 ripe pears
1 tbsp lemon juice
2 avocados
75 g/ 3 oz Dolcelatte cheese
115 g/ 4 oz wild rocket
50 g/ 2 oz walnut halves, roughly broken
4 tbsp Italian-style salad dressing

Quarter the pears and remove cores, then place in a bowl and sprinkle with lemon juice. Quarter the avocados and remove the stones. Peel and slice each quarter lengthways into 3 slices. Arrange the pears and avocados on a plate. Sprinkle with Dolcelatte, rocket and walnuts, then drizzle over the dressing.

Avocado is the one fruit that contains fat, and the flesh can be used like butter to spread on bread. This used to be called 'midshipman's butter' because it could be used at sea when ordinary butter went rancid. Eating too many avocados is fattening, but the fats they contain are the mainly 'good' unsaturated kind, both mono- and polyunsaturated. They reduce the cholesterol level in the blood (good for the heart) and provide plenty of antioxidants. They also have a reputation for protecting you against cancer, particularly of the bowel – just what is needed in diverticulitis.

There are over five hundred kinds of avocado, to suit different climates. In Britain, not one of the sunniest places, there are just two favourites: the smooth-skinned, green Fuerte and the darker, knobbly Hass variety. When they are ripe the skins become almost purple and give slightly when you press them, without going soft. Ripe avocados will keep for several days in the fridge, but if they are cut open the flesh quickly discolours unless the exposed part is immediately brushed with lemon juice or briefly held under the cold tap.

## Fruity Chicken Curry
8 skinless chicken fillets, cubed
4 tbsp malt vinegar
2 tbsp medium curry powder
1 tbsp ground cumin
1 tbsp ground coriander
$1/4$ tbsp turmeric
1 clove garlic, crushed
1 cm / $1/2$ inch ginger, crushed
4 tbsp brown sugar
4 tbsp sunflower oil
2 large onions, finely chopped
175 g / 6 oz ready-to-eat dried apricots, chopped
2 cloves
$1/4$ tsp peppercorns

In a large bowl mix together the vinegar, curry powder, cumin, coriander, turmeric, garlic, ginger and sugar. Mix in the chicken and leave to marinate in the refrigerator for 30 minutes. Heat the oil in a large pan add to this the onions and fry until they start to turn golden brown. Add the cloves and peppercorns and colour for 30 seconds. Add the chicken and marinade to the pan with the onions and simmer for 30-35 minutes or until the chicken is cooked thoroughly. Add the apricots, cover and cook for a further 15 minutes.

Serve with pilau rice, naan bread and a tomato and red onion salad. Serves 8.

Alternatively, instead of coconut milk and diced coconut, ordinary coconut milk with a handful of desiccated coconut mixed in works very well, and the fruit can be replaced with fresh or canned mango and pineapple.

## Watermelon with Lime Syrup
25 g / 1 oz caster sugar, less if you like it sharp
1 kg / 2 lb 4 oz watermelon
1 tbsp finely shredded mint
grated rind and juice of 1 lime

Put the lime juice and sugar in a small saucepan over a low heat to dissolve the sugar, then boil to a syrupy consistency. Pour into a jug and cool for 20 minutes, then refrigerate for an hour, or better still overnight. Peel the watermelon, then remove and discard the seeds. Cut the flesh into bite-size chunks, catching the juice in a bowl. Sprinkle the watermelon chunks with the mint and toss together lightly. Add the reserved melon juice to the chilled syrup and pour over the melon. Sprinkle with grated lime rind. Serve immediately: a heatwave special!

## Fruit Crumble
450 g/ 1 lb cooking apples, rhubarb, gooseberries, damsons, plums, blackberries, redcurrants or blackcurrants
75-100 g/ 3-4 oz granulated sugar to taste
175 g/ 6 oz flour
75 g/ 3 oz butter
50 g/ 2 oz caster sugar (or demerara if using a microwave)
Prepare the fruit and put into a 2 pt ovenproof dish in layers with the granulated sugar, keeping to the minimum of sugar that is needed for taste. Sift the flour into a bowl and rub in the butter until it resembles fine breadcrumbs. Stir in the caster or demerara sugar. Sprinkle the crumble thickly and evenly over the fruit. Press down lightly with the palm of your hand and smooth the top with a knife. Bake at 190°C/375°F/gas mark 5 for about 15 minutes, until the top is lightly brown. Serve with natural yoghurt, soured cream or custard.

This is a wonderfully variable and nutritious dish, bursting with vitamins, minerals and plant proteins.

## Oatie Fruit Crumble
Follow the recipe for Fruit Crumble, but for the crumble topping substitute wholemeal flour, brown sugar and 25 g/ 1 oz porridge oats. The oats add flavour and fibre.

## Crispy Lemon Crumble
Use the Fruit Crumble recipe, but add the grated rind of 1 lemon and 2 tbsp of crushed cornflakes to the topping.

## Ginger Fruit Crumble
Follow the same recipe, but for the topping use demerara sugar instead of caster and add 1 tsp ground ginger.

## Hot Apricot Soufflé
1 can (398 g/ 14 oz) apricot halves
$\frac{1}{2}$ tsp grated lemon rind

1 tsp lemon juice
1 tbsp granulated sugar
4 egg whites
$\frac{1}{4}$ tsp cream of tartar
1 tsp cornflour

Drain the apricots and pat dry with a paper towel. In a blender, pureé the apricots, lemon rind, lemon juice and sugar. In a large bowl, beat the egg whites and cream of tartar until stiff peaks form. Sift the cornflour over the egg whites and fold in with a metal spoon. Add about a quarter of the beaten egg whites to the apricot mixture and mix until just combined, then add the remaining egg whites and fold together. Pour into an ungreased 3-pt soufflé dish. Bake at 180°C/350°F/gas mark 4 for 30-35 minutes until puffed and golden brown. Serve immediately. Serves 4.

## Citrus Salad
2 limes, peeled and thinly sliced
1 small lemon, peeled and segmented
4 sweet oranges, peeled and coarsely chopped
4 mandarins, peeled and coarsely chopped
23 grapefruits, peeled and coarsely chopped
1 tsp granulated sugar
1 tsp Angostura bitters
3 tbsp sparkling mineral water
1 bunch of fresh mint and shredded mint leaves to garnish

Using a potato peeler, scrape wafer-thin slivers from the prepared fruit. With a pestle and mortar, crush the slivers with the sugar to release the highly-flavoured oils. Combine with the Angostura bitters and mineral waters and set aside. Plunge the bunch of fresh mint, tied with a piece of thread, in and out of boiling water, then straight into the bowl of fruit. Cover and chill for 2 hours. Remove the bunch of mint before serving and stir in the shredded mint leaves to garnish. Serves 6.

Wonderfully refreshing and full of vitamin C in particular! Good if you feel a cold coming on. If you find it too sharp, add a tablespoon of honey, slightly warmed so that it mixes in easily.

## Summer Fruits with Honeyed Oat Topping
4 apricots, pitted and halved
4 strawberries, hulled and halved
1 dsp clear honey
1 tbsp Greek yoghurt

1 tbsp medium rolled oats
1 tbsp roasted almonds

Put the apricots and strawberries in a bowl. Add the Greek yoghurt and honey and sprinkle the oats and almonds on top. Serves 1.

This is a low GI dish, providing 9 g protein, 36 g carbohydrate, and 12 g fat, amounting to 275 kcals.

## Frosted Fruit Mould
135 g/ 4¾ oz packet of lemon jelly
75 ml/ 5 tbsp boiling water
150 ml/¼ pt apricot purée made from stewed or canned apricots, fairly
    thick
2 tsp grated lemon rind
150 g/ 5 oz natural yoghurt
16 black grapes in pairs
1 egg white, lightly beaten
3 tbsp caster sugar

Put the jelly and boiling water in a pan and stand over a very low heat until the jelly dissolves. Pour into a measuring jug and make up to 300 ml/½ pt with cold water. Stir in the fruit purée and lemon rind. Leave until cold but still liquid, then gradually beat into the yoghurt. When evenly combined, transfer to a 1 pt jelly mould, rinsed first with cold water. Chill for at least 2 hours in the fridge. Before serving, frost the grapes by dipping in beaten egg white then tossing in caster sugar. Turn the jelly mould out onto a plate and surround with the frosted grapes. Serves 4.

## Fresh Peaches with Banana Cream Whip
1 egg white
1 large banana, mashed
1 tbsp icing sugar
1 tsp lemon juice
350 g/ 12 oz sliced fresh peaches or tinned peaches in natural juice

In a small bowl, beat the egg white until foamy. Add the banana, icing sugar and lemon juice and beat until the mixture forms stiff peaks. Spoon the peaches into individual dishes and top with banana cream. Serves 4.

A quick, low-calorie family dessert which can be served on sliced plums or apricots or various berries. It is best made an hour or less before serving because it darkens on standing and does not look so attractive.

## Fruit Bubble Cake (Bublanina)

125 g/ 4 oz butter
150 g/ 5 oz caster sugar
3 eggs
250 g/ 8 oz plain flour
150 ml/ ¼ pt milk
lemon rind
vanilla essence
1 kg/ 2 lb dried fruit
icing sugar for dusting

Separate the eggs and beat the egg whites until stiff. Warm the butter slightly, then cream with the sugar. Add the egg yolks and beat until the mixture is thick and creamy. Add spoonfuls of flour and milk alternately with a little grated lemon rind and vanilla essence. Fold in the stiffly whipped egg whites. Pile into a baking tin so that the layer is about 1 inch thick. Dot with the washed and stoned fruit cherries are the best. Bake in a slow to moderate oven until the surface is a light golden colour. Dust with icing sugar before serving.

## Calories and GI Index in fruits per 25 g/ 1 oz

| | | |
|---|---|---|
| Apple: | 13 kcal | low GI |
| Apple juice: | 43 kcal | low GI |
| Apricot, fresh: | 8 kcal | medium GI |
| Apricots, canned: | 18 kcal | medium GI |
| Apricots, dried: | 53 kcal | low GI |
| Avocado: | 54 kcal | low GI |
| Banana: | 26 kcal | medium GI |
| Blackberries: | 7 kcal | low GI |
| Blueberries: | 8 kcal | low GI |
| Cantaloupe melon: | 19 kcal | medium GI |
| Cherries: | 11 kcal | low GI |
| Cranberry juice: | 51 kcal | medium GI |
| Dates, fresh: | 31 kcal | high GI |
| Dates, dried: | 77 kcal | high GI |
| Figs, fresh: | 12 kcal | medium GI |
| Figs, dried: | 65 kcal | medium GI |
| Fruit cocktail canned in juice: | 8 kcal | medium GI |
| Fruit cocktail canned in syrup: | 16 kcal | medium GI |
| Grapefruit: | 9 kcal | low GI |
| Grapes, white: | 16 kcal | low GI |

| | | |
|---|---|---|
| Grapes, red: | 16 kcal | medium GI |
| Kiwi fruit: | 12 kcal | low GI |
| Lemons: | 4 kcal | low GI |
| Limes: | 2 kcal | low GI |
| Mandarin: | 11 kcal | low GI |
| Mango: | 18 kcal | medium GI |
| Olives: | 34 kcal | low GI |
| Oranges: | 7 kcal | low GI |
| Papaya: | 30 kcal | medium GI |
| Peaches, fresh: | 8 kcal | low GI |
| Peaches, canned in juice: | 11 kcal | medium GI |
| Peaches, canned in syrup: | 16 kcal | medium GI |
| Pears, fresh: | 12 kcal | low GI |
| Pears, canned in juice: | 9 kcal | low GI |
| Pears, canned in syrup: | 14 kcal | medium GI |
| Pineapple, fresh: | 12 kcal | medium GI |
| Pineapple, canned in juice: | 13 kcal | medium GI |
| Pineapple, canned in syrup: | 18 kcal | medium GI |
| Plums: | 10 kcal | low GI |
| Prunes: | 38 kcal | low GI |
| Raisins: | 78 kcal | medium GI |
| Raspberries: | 7 kcal | low GI |
| Satsumas: | 11 kcal | low GI |
| Strawberries: | 8 kcal | low GI |
| Sultanas: | 79 kcal | medium GI |
| Tomatoes, fresh: | 5 kcal | low GI |
| Tomatoes, canned: | 5 kcal | low GI |
| Watermelon, with skin: | 5 kcal | high GI |
| Watermelon, peeled: | 9 kcal | high GI |

# Herbs and Spices

Herbs and spices add a touch of magic, transforming a dish that was dull and unexciting, spicing it up so that it tickles your taste buds and sparks off your appetite. All this comes without any time-consuming or complicated cookery. The secret lies in a pinch of spice or a leaf or seed from a fresh or dried herb. The magic floods through every mouthful of food, instilling a flavour and most importantly a scent, from France to Arabia, the Far East to simple Britain. They are ideal for experimenting with new dishes on a small scale and cheaply. Among the best-loved and most often used herbs and spices are chopped chives with their mild oniony taste and decorative value, or freshly peeled and chopped ginger root, which literally 'gingers up' a cake, a biscuit or a pudding.

Even if your garden is only a window box, you can 'grow your own food' on a miniature scale with herbs – even children can manage to grow mustard and cress. Mint flourishes anywhere. Another advantage of herbs is that you can keep them in fresh condition by chopping them and packing a teaspoonful into each ice-cube tray, topping them up with water and freezing. You can use them a cube at a time: they look limp but the flavour is retained. For herbs to sprinkle on a dish, for instance as a garnish, it is better to freeze-dry them. They can be stored in little plastic bags or pots for use when needed. Thyme, chives and oregano freeze-dry particularly well.

## Common Herbs

| | |
|---|---|
| *Bay leaves* | can be used fresh or dried, and are especially good boiled with milk puddings and custards. |
| *Basil* | too, can be used either fresh or dried, with almost anything: eggs, fish, meat, pasta, tomatoes, etc. It improves most sauces and salads. |
| *Chives* | pep up eggs, cheese, soups and sauces. |
| *Dill* | leaves are best known for pickling cucumber, but are excellent in salads or sprinkled on cooked meat and hot or cold fish dishes, especially prawns. The seeds have a different, stronger taste, a little like caraway. They give flavour to boring boiled potatoes and can be cooked with pork. |
| *Garlic* | is used with almost everything in France, the Mediterranean |

countries and all over Asia. It has a strong taste and smell, lasting for hours on the breath all right so long as everyone shares the same meal. It has a wonderful reputation for health: for the heart and blood pressure, the chest and the digestive system. Not everyone likes it, however, nor enjoys noticing when someone else has been eating it. Nevertheless it is probably the most popular adjunct to a main meal. It is at its best when fresh, when the cloves are plump and hard, and crushed so as to give the maximum taste and aroma.

*Mint* grows like a weed and spreads like one, with no trouble. It has a refreshing flavour that enhances that of both savoury and sweet foods. Mint sauce is a must with lamb in Britain, but is an agreeable addition, chopped, to stews, meatballs and chicken, and sprinkled over vegetables.

*Oregano* and Marjoram: oregano, or wild marjoram, goes very well with eggs, cheese, tomatoes, mushrooms, fish and minced pork or beef in a wide variety of dishes. Cultivated English marjoram has a similar but milder, sweeter taste. It goes well with liver and, unexpectedly, with rice pudding, used sparingly.

*Parsley* makes a pleasant-looking and tasting garnish, and is an excellent source of iron.

*Rosemary* is available, fresh, all the year round. It improves roasts such as chicken, lamb or pork, and most stews and casseroles, and makes an elegant garnish. Boil a sprig with the milk for its delicate flavour to permeate sweet milk puddings and sauces.

*Tarragon* is another popular herb because it is so versatile. Chopped finely and used sparingly it brings out the taste of chicken, vegetables, salads, cheese and fish. It also transforms thick soups and creamy sauces and improves the flavour of wine vinegar.

*Thyme* was already in use for flavouring by the ancient Greeks. It has a strong flavour and aroma that makes it suitable for slow-cooking meat, poultry and game casseroles and stews. Sprigs of thyme introduced into incisions in a joint of lamb before roasting make it smell delicious and taste just as good.

*Sage* in sage and onion stuffing, reminiscent of Christmas and turkey, but it is equally tasty with veal and pork and in beef stews, as well as with quite different light cheese or egg dishes.

Herbs and spices are often presented in sauces, jellies, relishes, chutneys, pickles, marinades and other accompaniments that make all the difference to ordinary dishes. They are like the jewellery that brings a touch of glamour to a simple dress.

## Spices

| | |
|---|---|
| *Chilli* | powder is made from red chillies and varies in its flavour and how hot it is, partly because other spices are often included with the chillies. It provides the basis for curry, and is well-known in the Mexican dish 'chilli con carne', that is with meat. A pinch of ground chilli livens up a creamy soup or an egg dish, but it is important to use it sparingly. |
| *Cardamom* | seeds, like chillies, are an important spice in curry and are both pungent and aromatic, so only a very little is required. The seeds are removed from their pods and ground finely. They are useful for adding flavour to dishes, whether roast, minced or casseroled, and sauces. They give a new pleasure in creamy puddings and ice-cream. |
| *Cinnamon* | like cardamom, enhances the flavour of either savoury or sweet dishes. It is especially popular with apple pies and cakes in England. In other countries it is highly-valued as an adjunct to chicken and lamb casseroles, which can be rather bland, and it is also good with roasts, especially duck. Usually it is sold ready-ground, but is also available as strips of bark. |
| *Cayenne* | pepper is extremely hot – beware! A tiny pinch is enough to liven up an egg dish or a cheese sauce. It is made by grinding red chilli pepper. |
| *Coriander* | seeds provide a mild aromatic spice that has been used in cooking for more than two thousand years, and more recently in pickling. The seeds are coarsely ground and used with roast and stewed meats, chicken, and baked fish. The seeds can be planted and the leaves used; these have a quite different, stronger taste. They enhance the flavour of salads and, chopped roughly and thrown in just before serving, transform a stew or a curry. They also improve a sauce. |
| *Cumin* | seeds are an important ingredient in curries, and although they are not used much in European cooking, their powerful flavour imprints itself on lamb stew, roast sand meatballs. |

| | |
|---|---|
| *Ginger* | is a popular flavouring and comes in several forms: ground, crystallized, or the bare root. Crystallized ginger is used in cakes, biscuits and other sweets, while the root is used in savoury dishes to give them a bite'. |
| *Green chilli* | is flavourful and sharp, but be careful to remove all the little seeds to avoid being burned! Try cautiously adding small amounts of finely chopped chilli to any dish you have at hand – it may be miraculously successful – or wipe a grilled steak with a broken piece of chilli instead of using freshly ground black pepper. |
| *Nutmeg* | is an old-fashioned spice that blends comfortably with both sweet and savoury dishes, in a gentle way. It goes with creamed potatoes and swedes, creamy stews and sauces, cream cheese and, unexpectedly, spinach. It is best to use a whole nutmeg and grate what you need freshly. It is possible to get acclimatised to this (or any other) spice and add increasing quantities to a daily smoothie, milk drink etc. Too much nutmeg can cause an irregular heartbeat and larger quantities could be hallucinogenic and may cause nightmares. |
| *Paprika* | is a red pepper, ground finely, but not a hot as cayenne or chilli so it can be used freely. It gives everything an attractive red colour and peps up sauces, stews and chicken, fish, egg and cheese dishes. |
| *Turmeric* | is related to ginger, and ground to a bright yellow powder. It is used in pickles, chutney and curry powders. It is good in rice dishes and also used sparingly in white sauce, soups and egg dishes. Recent research has revealed turmeric's potential cancer fighting action. |

## Recipes

**Fresh Mint Sauce**
3 tbsp granulated sugar
75 ml/ 2½ fl oz cider vinegar
60 ml/ 2 fl oz water
7 ml/ 1½ tsp cornflour
20 g/ ⅔ oz tightly packed, finely chopped fresh mint leaves

Combine sugar, vinegar, water and cornflour in a small pan. Bring to the boil over a medium heat, stirring constantly. Stir in the mint and simmer for 3 minutes, then transfer to a sauce boat and let it stand for 30 minutes for the flavour to develop. Will keep in the fridge for up to two months.

## Red or Green Pepper Jelly
900g/ 2 lb granulated sugar
3 medium-sized red or green peppers, finely chopped
375 ml/ 12 fl oz white vinegar
170-ml bottle of liquid pectin

Combine the sugar, peppers and vinegar, stir and bring to the boil. Boil over a medium heat for 15 minutes, skimming off the foam. Remove from the heat and blend in the pectin, stirring for 2 minutes. Pour into sterilized jars, leaving 15 mm/ ¼ inch space at the top. Seal with paraffin wax and cover with lids. Store in a cool, dry place.

## Mint and Pea Soup
75 g/ 3 oz butter or spread
1 small onion, roughly chopped
12 cloves of garlic, chopped
large handful of fresh mint leaves
450 g/ 1 lb shelled fresh or frozen peas
1 l / 2 pt chicken stock
150 ml / ¼ pt natural yoghurt
juice of a small lemon
salt and black pepper to taste

Melt the butter and add the onion, garlic, mint (save a little for a garnish), peas and stock. Bring to the boil, cover and simmer gently until the peas and onions are tender, about 10 – 15 minutes. Leave to cool and blend in a liquidizer until smooth. Add the yoghurt, and stir in the lemon juice very gradually. Season. Serve either chilled in the fridge or reheated; garnish with mint leaves.

## Duck with Olives and Cinnamon
4 breast and wing or leg joints of duck
2 tsp ground cinnamon
1 tbsp olive or sunflower oil
2 cloves of garlic, crushed or chopped finely
5075 g/ 2-3 oz black olives, stoned and chopped
black pepper and a trace of salt
juice of 2 oranges
150 ml/ ¼ pt water
25 g/ 1 oz flaked almonds (optional)

a little chopped parsley to garnish

Heat the oven to the highest setting. Cut the breast joints in half and rub all over with cinnamon (the top flavour for the dish). Heat the oil and fry the pieces of duck until just browned on both sides. Stir in the garlic and fry for a minute more. Arrange the pieces of duck in a casserole dish. Sprinkle the olives over the duck together with seasoning. Pour in the orange juice and water. Cover and bring to simmering point in the oven for around 20 minutes, then turn down to 180°C/350°F/gas mark 4 for 45 minutes to 1 hour. Check the tenderness of the duck with a knife. Pour the juices from the casserole into a saucepan and skim off as much fat as you can. Boil the juices at the highest setting until reduced and slightly thickened, about 8-10 minutes. Pour the sauce over the duck, cover and keep warm. Just before serving, fry the flaked almonds until browning, then sprinkle over the duck. Finally scatter the chopped parsley over the top. Serves 4, with rice and a green salad.

### Lamb's Liver with Paprika and Cumin
450 g/ 1 lb lamb's or, better still, calf's liver, cut into thin slices
2 tbsp wine vinegar
5-6 tbsp olive or sunflower oil
4 tbsp milk
black pepper, trace of salt
2-3 onions, sliced thinly
2 cloves garlic, crushed or chopped finely
2 tsp paprika
2 tsp ground cumin
handful of fresh chopped parsley for garnish
wedges of lemon for garnish

Put the sliced liver into a shallow, ovenproof dish. Mix the vinegar with 2 tbsp of oil and the milk, season and pour over the liver. Cover the dish and leave in a cool place to marinate for several hours. Heat 3 more tbsp of oil and fry the onion gently until soft. Add the garlic and spices and cook for a minute or two. Add a little more oil if necessary and turn up the heat. Put in the marinated liver and toss for 2-3 minutes no longer. Transfer to a serving dish, sprinkle with chopped parsley and garnish with lemon to squeeze over the liver when eating. Serve with boiled potato and parsnip, mashed together with butter, a little milk, black pepper and a grating of nutmeg and a green vegetable or salad leaves. Serves 4.

## Breast of Turkey or Chicken Coriander

450 g/ 1 lb boned turkey or chicken
2.5 cm/ 1-inch piece of fresh green ginger or ½ tsp ground ginger
2 tsp coriander seed
2 cloves of garlic
2 tbsp tomato puree
juice of 1 lemon
3 tbsp sunflower or other cooking oil
black pepper, trace of salt
1 small head of celery, sliced in rings
150 ml/ 5 fl oz natural yoghurt
100 g/ 4 oz cashew nuts

Preheat the oven to 180°C/350°F/gas mark 4. Skin the chicken breasts and cut them across in medium slices. Grind the coriander seed using a pestle and mortar. Cut the skin off the fresh ginger, peel the cloves of garlic and finely chop both together. Put in a mixing bowl with the ground coriander, tomato puṙe, lemon juice and 2 tbsp of the oil. Season and stir in the sliced chicken and celery. Cover the bowl with a cloth and leave to marinate in the fridge overnight. Transfer the mixture to a casserole dish. Stand for 30 minutes at room temperature, then cover and cook for 50-60 minutes. Stir in the yoghurt and put back in the oven for a further 5-10 minutes. Finally, fry the cashew nuts until golden and scatter over the chicken or turkey. Serves 4.

# Breakfasts, Elevenses and Nightcaps

## Wake-up Call for Your Colon

First thing in the morning drink a mugful of hot tea, coffee, diluted lemon juice (PLJ) or plain water. This clears your digestive system ready for action. A plain biscuit, Rich Tea or similar, gives your blood sugar a lift to start the day's bodily activities.

A good – read 'substantial' – breakfast has long been regarded as the mainspring of the day's nourishment. It should be enough to keep you going during the day without recourse to junky snacks or the pernicious habit of grazing. A study on schoolchildren showed that those who had a 'proper' breakfast performed better at school – intellectually, at games and in having fewer infections. Among adults, those who skip breakfast – often with the idea of slimming – actually put on more weight, with biscuits, chocolate bars, and other snacks.

Breakfast recipes should be quick and easy to prepare and adaptable for all ages, as none of us has time to spare in the morning. Today's typical morning meal is cereal with milk, toast, spread and marmalade or honey. It needs a whole apple, orange or banana or a couple of tablespoons of stewed fruit to increase the proportion of fibre sufficiently to signal to the colon to empty the waste. Hot cereal or hot milk on the cereal peps up its stimulating effect as with other hot, cooked meals.

### Winter breakfasts
Porridge
600 ml/ 1 pt of water, or half water and half skimmed milk
100 g/ 4 oz rolled oats

Cook the oats and water in a saucepan or in the microwave until the porridge is the thickness you like. Serve with skimmed milk and sugar or honey, or a sprinkle of salt if you preferred. Balance with stewed or raw fruit.

Oat bran, unlike wheat bran, reduces the amount of cholesterol in the blood and is recommended by the British Heart Foundation.

Readybrek, a hot oat cereal, doubles for porridge but only requires the stirring in of a cupful of boiling water or skimmed milk to 6 heaped dessertspoons (40 g) of the powder or the same quantities but starting with cold water or milk for 2 ½ minutes in the microwave at full heat.

Wheat cereals, such as Weetabix or Shredded Wheat, with very hot water or milk also make an instant warming and nourishing meal. Extra fibre can be introduced by adding stewed or fresh fruit, or dried fruits such as apricots or prunes soaked overnight and then heated in the microwave. Note, however, that the process of flaking cereals releases more sugar and increases the calorie-count.

## Eggs
The versatile egg may be boiled, poached, coddled or scrambled and served with toast, olive oil spread and marmalade or honey, and an apple, orange or banana. Eggs may be fried as a Sunday treat for men, as their bodies can cope with a little more fat.

Eggs contain several valuable nutrients but, in excess, too much fat. Harvard research studies have shown that moderate egg consumption, up to one a day does not increase heart disease risk in healthy individuals. Yolks have a lot of cholesterol but also heart protective nutrients such as protein, vitamins B12 and D, riboflavin and folate. Diabetics should limit their intake to 2 or 3 eggs per week. They contain lecithin, which helps the liver break down fats, and sulphur, which helps it deal with alcohol and various toxins.

## Toast Dishes
*Sardines* on toast provide protein, fat and calcium a guard against osteoporosis, and a provider of the essential omega-3 oil. Pilchards are similar.
*Cheese* on toast (Welsh rarebit) with grilled tomatoes and sliced apple. Buck rarebit is the same as Welsh rarebit but with a poached or fried egg on top: watch your fats for the rest of the day and go for fruit, vegetables and fibre.

## Ham and Tomato Scramble
1 slice of lean ham
a handful of mushrooms
2 tomatoes, chopped
2 eggs
1 tbs skimmed milk
olive oil for cooking

Arrange the ham, mushrooms and tomatoes on a dish. Beat together the eggs and skimmed milk and pour over the dish. Cook under the grill for 3 minutes.

Like dairy and other animal-sourced protein, ham contains all the essential amino-acids as opposed to vegetable protein.

## Summer Breakfasts
With all of these have 2-3 Ryvita biscuits spread with Marmite, or one only spread with honey. Dark rye biscuits provide more fibre than ordinary Ryvita or wheat crispbreads such as Macvita.

## Berry Mix Smoothie
25 g/ 1 oz blueberries, blackcurrants or redcurrants
85 g/ 3 oz raspberries, strawberries or loganberries
1 tsp runny honey
150 ml/ ¼ pt yoghurt
beetroot, pear and spinach juice
1 beetroot, trimmed, peeled and chopped
1 pear, peeled, cored and chopped
25 g/ 1 oz spinach leaves

Process all ingredients in a blender or liquidizer. This drink stimulates the digestive and water systems for a clean start. Beetroot in particular boosts the action of the liver and the bowels, while pears, like apples, contain pectin, a fibre that slows the rate of sugar release from the fruit.

An alternative combination is apple, carrot and cucumber juice, full of antioxidants and soluble fibre.

## Fresh Fruit Muesli
115 g/ 4 oz apples, blackberries, strawberries, plums, apricots, cherries, or bananas, chopped or sliced
1 tbsp porridge oats, soaked in 1 tbsp water
handful of chopped hazelnuts

Mix all the ingredients together, finishing with the hazelnuts. Serve with soya milk or skimmed milk.

## Dried Fruit and Nut Muesli
115 g/ 4 oz porridge oats
85 g/ 3 oz each of shelled pecans, almonds, brazil nuts and hazelnuts, chopped or flaked
85 g/ 3 oz raisins
85 g/ 3 oz each of dried figs, apricots and peaches, chopped
25 g/ 1 oz sunflower seeds

Mix the ingredients together in a bowl. Serve with apple juice, soya milk or plain yoghurt.

Walnuts provide the amino acid tryptophan which the brain cells convert into the neurotransmitter serotonin needed to combat depression and maintain cheerfulness, they can be used instead of other nuts. Bananas also have a perk-up effect, but of course do not keep like nuts.

Dried fruit muesli can be prepared in larger quantities than the fresh fruit type, and kept in an airtight container until needed.

## Sunshine Bars

150 ml/ ¼ pt milk
100 g/ 4 oz dried dates, stoned and chopped
175 g/ 6 oz wholemeal self-raising flour
2.5 ml/ ½ tsp baking powder
2.5 ml/ ½ tsp ground cinnamon
1 egg, beaten
50 g/ 2 oz butter, melted
grated rind and chopped flesh of 1 orange or 1 grapefruit

Grease and line an 18 cm/ 7-inch square tin. Warm the milk, add the dates and stand for 15 minutes. Mix the flour, baking powder and cinnamon in a bowl. Beat the egg, melted butter and orange rind into the milk. Stir in the dry ingredients and orange flesh and mix well. Spoon into the baking tin and bake at 160°C/325°F/gas mark 3 for 40 minutes or until golden brown. Cut into fingers when cool. This recipe makes 10 fingers. It contains no added sugar. Serve with stewed apple, plums or rhubarb, or fresh fruit. It will keep in an airtight tin for a few days only.

## Bran Muffins

50 g/ 2 oz bran
300 ml/ ½ pt milk
50 g/ 2 oz caster sugar
50 g/ 2 oz butter or spread
1 egg, beaten
50 g/ 2 oz raisins
100 g/ 4 oz wholemeal flour
15 ml/ 1 tbsp baking powder
pinch of salt

Soak the bran in milk for 10 minutes. Cream together the sugar and butter until light and fluffy. Beat together the egg, raisins, bran and milk. Sift together the flour, baking powder and a pinch of salt and fold into the bran mixture. Grease 6 muffin tins or use paper cases. Bake in a pre-heated oven at 19°C/375°F/gas mark 5 for 15-20 minutes or until a toothpick inserted into the centre of a muffin comes out clean. Serve warm with bananas or other fresh fruit.

The bran and the fibre in the fruit is stimulating to the colon, and there are also vitamin C and niacin to ward off infections.

## More Breakfasts

1   ½ melon or grapefruit, 125 g/ 5 oz low fat fruit yoghurt, 3 oatcakes with a scrape of olive oil spread, 150 ml/ ¼ pt orange juice or whole orange in segments, wholewheat cereal (e.g. Shreddies, Weetabix) and sliced banana with semi-skimmed milk, wholemeal toast with peanut butter.

2   Croissant, strawberry jam, 125 g/ 5 oz carton of cottage cheese or half-fat crème fraîche and a large apple.

3   3 plums, 1 small, sliced banana, topped with 2 tbsp plain, low-fat yoghurt and 1 tbsp muesli.

4   Poached egg, slice of wholemeal toast, grilled tomato and mushroom, orange juice.

5   2 Weetabix, 150 ml/ ¼ pt skimmed milk, 1 orange, 1 §-inch cube of mild Cheddar cheese.

6   4-5 dried apricots, soaked overnight with a bowl of Shreddies or Cornflakes with skimmed milk, 1-2 oatcakes.

## Fish Brunch

100 g/ 3½ oz brown rice
few strands of saffron
300 g/ 10½ oz smoked haddock fillets
1 large onion
1 crushed garlic clove (optional)
2 tomatoes, chopped
115 g/ 4 oz French beans, chopped
115 g/ 4 oz sweetcorn
2 tbsp olive oil
150 ml/ 5 fl oz fish stock
150 ml/ 5 fl oz milk
1 tbsp fresh coriander

Boil the rice and saffron until tender. Add the other ingredients, mix and cook for 25 minutes.

The rice husks contain B vitamins and fibre, slowing the release of starch and sugar into the bloodstream. Vitamin C, other antioxidants and protein (with all the essential amino acids) are provided by the fish, milk, etc.

**Pancakes**
125 g / 4 oz wholemeal flour
1 egg
300 ml / ½ pt skimmed milk
1 tbsp vegetable oil or melted butter
juice and wedges of 1 orange or 1 lemon

Sift the flour into a bowl and break in the egg. Gradually add half the milk, beating to make a smooth batter. Pour in the remaining milk and beat until quite smooth. Stir in the melted butter or oil, heating gently. When the pan and butter are hot, add 3 tbsp of batter, tilting the pan to cover the base. Cook until the batter moves freely and is turning golden, turn and cook other side. Sprinkle with sugar and lemon or orange juice. Roll the pancake over a fork with wedges of fruit at each turn. Repeat until all the batter is used, stacking the pancakes on a large plate, covered and standing over gently simmering water.

Other fruit can be used, for instance thinly sliced apple, plum, peach, kiwi fruit, strawberries, blackberries or raspberries. The result is a hot dish containing antioxidant-laden fresh fruit.

## Other Breakfast Ideas

Breakfast is such an important meal, providing half your day's nourishment on average. Missing out on breakfast leads to big elevenses and other mainly sweet carbohydrate snacks. This can be the equivalent of two cups of sugar daily.

1    150 ml / ¼ pt unsweetened orange juice or an orange, 2 slices of granary bread, spread with 2 tsp ricotta cheese, and 2 tsp of all-fruit conserve, for instance blackberry.
2    1 boiled egg, 2 rye crispbreads topped with yeast extract, ½ a grapefruit, smoothie made from 150 ml / ¼ pt skimmed milk and 2 handfuls of berries (e.g. blackberries, blueberries or raspberries).
3    2 rashers of back bacon, trimmed of all fat, grilled mushroom, grilled tomato, 100 g / 3 ½ oz canned baked beans and 1 slice of granary toast.
4    Bowl of porridge made with 75 g / 3 oz rolled oats with 25 g / 1 oz sultanas and half an apple, finely chopped and all mixed well

together, and 150 ml/¹⁄₄ pt unsweetened orange or grapefruit juice
5       1 scrambled egg, 2-3 grilled mushrooms, a slice of granary toast
        with 25 g/ 1 oz butter and 150 ml/ ¹⁄₄ pt apple juice.
6       1 mango, 100 g/ 3 oz Cheshire cheese, 3 dark rye crispbreads and
        decaffeinated tea or coffee with skimmed milk.

## Some other healthy choices for breakfast are:

- Orange or other fresh fruit: trace of fat, 62 calories instead of croissant: 12 g fat, 235 calories.
- Wholegrain cereal: trace of fat, 93 calories instead of fried egg and bacon: 18 g fat, 241 calories. Bacon traditionally accompanies eggs at breakfast, but is not a healthy choice. It is high in saturated fat, salt and nitrates, all of them best avoided.
- Stewed prunes or dried fruit salad go well with low-fat yoghurt, or a low-sugar cereal: trace of fat, 90 calories instead of coffee with cream: 3 g fat, 28 calories.

## Fat and Calorie Count in Breakfast Ingredients

|  | Grammes of fat | Calories |
|---|---|---|
| Orange juice ¹⁄₄ pt/ 150 ml | trace | 59 |
| Grapefruit ¹⁄₂ | trace | 93 |
| Melon ¹⁄₂ | trace | 90 |
| Low-fat fruit yoghurt 125 g/ 5 oz tub | 2 | 131 |
| Sliced banana, 1 | trace | 105 |
| Wholewheat cereal, 50 g/ 2 oz | trace | 165 |
| Bran Flakes, 50 g/ 2 oz | trace | 139 |
| Slice of white bread toast, 1 | trace | 76 |
| Slice of wholemeal toast | trace | 61 |
| Unsaturated margarine, 1 tsp/ 5 ml | 4 | 33 |
| Peanut butter, 1 tbsp/ 15 ml | 8 | 95 |
| Semi-skimmed milk, 300 ml/ ¹⁄₂ pt | 5 | 128 |

## How much? Servings Per Day
Milk and dairy products: adult 2, adolescent 34
Examples of 1 serving:
300 ml/ ¹⁄₂ pt milk
150 g/ 6 oz yoghurt

49 g / 1½ oz cheddar cheese

## Bread and cereals: 3-5, wholegrain preferred
Examples of 1 serving:
1 slice wholemeal bread
40 g / 1½ oz cooked cereal
40 g / 1½ oz ready-to-eat cereal
1 bread roll
1 tbsp cooked rice or pasta
Fruit and vegetables: 56, including at least 2 vegetable servings, cooked, raw or in their own juice, yellow or green

Examples of 1 serving:
100 g / 4 oz fruit, vegetable or juice
1 medium-size potato, carrot, tomato, peach, orange, banana or apple
Protein foods suitable for breakfast: 2-3

Examples of 1 serving:
1 or 2 eggs*
2 rashers bacon, back with fat trimmed off
2 sardines
50 g / 2 oz cheddar or Leicester cheese
75 g / 3 oz cottage cheese*
50 g / 2 oz nuts*
125 g / 5 oz peanut butter*
*Use only once a week because of high fat content.

## High-fibre Foods, Especially Important at Breakfast
- breakfast cereals (40 g / 1½ oz) especially bran type and wholegrain
- porridge
- baked beans
- wholemeal bread/toast
- fruit: apple, pear, banana, berries, orange, grapefruit, cantaloupe melon, dried apricots, prunes, figs, raisins
- nuts (peanuts, almonds, brazils, walnuts)

Eat 8-10 servings daily from the high-fibre list, and drink 8 glasses of water or the equivalent amount of liquid. The liquid is especially necessary to keep diverticular problems at bay.

## Elevenses
If you are one of those who has a very light breakfast or don't have time, a

mid-morning coffee break is a life-saver, but make it decaffeinated with skimmed or soya milk, and of course no sugar. Try to avoid artificial sweeteners cut down in small steps, if you must. A wholemeal scone and an apple, an orange or a banana is a better choice than a Danish pastry and strong coffee with cream full of fat and calories but short on fibre and vitamins. Other between-meal pick-me-ups (non-alcoholic) include:

- 4-5 dried apricots, 4-5 walnuts or hazelnuts, tea with skimmed milk
- slice of granary bread with 25 g/ 1 oz cottage cheese, fruit tea
- 125 g/ 5 oz carton of low-fat fruit yoghurt, 25 g/ 1 oz Edam cheese, 2 dark rye crispbreads, 6 white grapes
- raw carrot, 2 digestive biscuits
- pear, banana or apple and 25 g/ 1 oz dark chocolate (contains catechins, antioxidants which cancel out its high fat content)
- 3-4 celery sticks (good for high blood pressure) with peanut butter
- 2 wheat crispbreads topped with thin slices of cheddar cheese
- pack of 6 little breadsticks and soft cheese
- slice of toast and honey and an apple
- smoothie made with soya or skimmed milk, a yoghurt and a handful of blackberries or other soft fruit. Blueberries and cranberries guard against urinary infection and also help keep cholesterol levels low.

## Nightcaps

Your eating day starts with a stimulating cup of tea or coffee, fruit and a good lining to carry you through whatever life throws at you. This is all reversed at bedtime. You don't want a hefty or complex meal to digest when you are going to lie down and sleep for some hours. The ideal is a warm, milky drink, because the fat in it calms and slows down your digestive system and calcium soothes the nerves. This is enough to waft you into the land of dreamless slumber, but you need a little more nourishment to last your body until breakfast time. This can be in the form of malted milk Horlicks is the best-known or one or two sweet, plain biscuits.

### Oat Biscuits
100 g/ 4 oz low fat spread
100 g/ 4 oz brown sugar
1 tbsp golden syrup
100 g/ 4 oz self-raising or wholemeal flour
250 g/ 9 oz rolled oats
1 tsp bicarbonate of soda, dissolved in 4 tbsps nearly boiling water

Put all the ingredients together and mix into a stiff dough. Roll out. This is enough to make 40 biscuits. Cook in a moderate oven until they are brown around 15 minutes. These biscuits are gently sustaining at night or with elevenses. Oates are widely recognised soothers of the brain and nerves.

## Alcoholic Nightcaps

Many elderly people, especially men, swear by a nip of whisky as a nightcap. It can be enjoyable for those who like it and excellent helping them to drop off quickly. The snag is that by about 3 a.m. all the whisky has been metabolized and you wake up at this unfriendly hour feeling rather bleak or, if you took too big a dose to start with, a hangover. No one gets a hangover from Horlicks. It also sometimes helps to nibble a Rich Tea or other sweet, plain biscuit.

# Fish and Seafood

Cardiovascular (meaning *heart-artery*) disease kills 300,000 of us every year in Britain. You can cut down your chances of being one of them by adopting the lifestyle recommended by The British Heart Foundation. We all know the rules: be active, don't smoke, drink in moderation or less and, most importantly of all, watch what you eat. Choose a varied diet to include all the necessary vitamins and minerals, plenty of starch and fibre, but strict limitations on fat and care not to overindulge in sugary foods. For most of us this means eating *less* total fat, particularly saturated fats, and *more* fruit, vegetables, fish and wholegrain breads and vegetables.

Fat is the major factor and this shows up as the level of cholesterol in the blood. There are two kinds of cholesterol: high density lipoproteins (HDL) which are 'good', and low-density lipoproteins (LDL) which tend to clog the blood vessels. The most effective dietary trick for reducing your blood cholesterol is to cut down on the saturated fat in your food, most easily done by reducing your total fat intake, unsaturated as well as saturated.

**Common sources of fat are:**
- meat, and meat products such as sausages, pies and paṫs
- cereal products, biscuits, cakes and puddings
- fat spreads, margarine
- milk and milk products such as butter, cheese, cream, ice-cream
- vegetables, especially roast, fried or mashed potatoes
- sugar-laden foods that stimulate the liver into manufacturing body fat
- *most importantly*, fish and seafood 2 which contain the right sort of fat.

The omega-3 fatty acids in certain fish oils help to prevent the development of atherosclerosis, blockage of the arteries by cholesterol, with a danger of clotting. The helpful fatty fish include salmon, sardines, anchovies, pilchards, trout, herrings, mackerel and tuna. *Canned* tuna, however, although tasty and a useful low-calorie source of protein, does not reduce the harmful triglyceride fats in the blood.

The British Heart Foundation recommends eating a fish meal two or three times a week, describing it as 'an investment in the future, for your heart'.

## Types of Fat

*Saturated* fats are usually solid at room temperature. They are found in cheese, meat, chocolate, highly hydrogenated margarines and vegetable oils. A maximum of 10 per cent of our calorie intake should come from these fats. Monounsaturated and polyunsaturated fats are usually liquid at room temperature.

*Monounsaturated* fats include rapeseed, sunflower and peanut oils, and some spreads and margarines and are also found in cashews and avocavocados. Olive oil is unspoiled by cooking and does you no harm.

*Polyunsaturated* fats include sunflower, corn and soyabean oils, some spreads and margarines, and are found in almonds, hazelnuts and fish.

### Safety Switch
Choose:
- 1 glass of skimmed milk instead of 1 glass of full cream milk
- 25 g/ 1 oz grated Edam, mozzarella or low-fat cheese instead of cheddar
- 50 g/ 2 oz of cottage cheese instead of of cream cheese a saving of 20 g fat
- 120 g/ 4 oz chicken without skin instead of with skin
- bread with 1 tsp margarine or spread instead of 2 tsp
- salad with1 tbsp of low-fat mayonnaise instead of ordinary mayonnaise
- 1 pear or tomato instead of 1 avocado a saving of 30 g fat
- apple crisp with oatmeal topping instead of apple pie
- a currant bun instead of rich fruit cake

### Other tips:

- Use a mere scraping of butter, margarine, spread or oils, low-fat if possible, on toast, on vegetables, in sandwiches and especially in cooking.
- Use lemon juice or herbs on vegetables instead of butter, to bring out the flavour.
- Avoid frying and swap to grilling, baking, steaming, poaching or boiling.
- Roast meat on a rack, or sauté in a non-stick pan.
- When the meat is browned, spoon off all the fat.
- Sauté vegetables in 5 ml/ 1 tsp oil and 60 ml/ 2 fl oz oil. This method uses less fat than stir-frying.

Salmon Steaks with Watercress Sauce
4 salmon steaks, 2.5 cm /1-inch thick, 125 g/ 5 oz each
2 tsp lemon juice
freshly ground pepper
sprigs of watercress
For the sauce:
275 g/ 10 oz low-fat cottage cheese
60 g/ 2½ oz low-fat natural yoghurt
25 g/ 1 oz fresh watercress leaves, chopped
2 tbsp fresh parsley, chopped
1 tbsp fresh chives, chopped
2 tsp Parmesan cheese, grated

Lay the salmon on lightly oiled foil and sprinkle with lemon juice and pepper. Bake for about 15 minutes, until the fish is opaque and flakes easily with a fork. To make the sauce, combine the cottage cheese, yoghurt, watercress, parsley, chives and Parmesan in a blender or press through a sieve. Arrange the salmon on individual plates and garnish with sprigs of watercress. Serve the sauce separately. Serves 4.

## Watercress, Tuna and White Bean Salad
225 g/ 8 oz cucumber
3 tomatoes
1 x 410 g can cannellini beans, drained
1 x 200 g can tuna chunks in spring water, drained
2 tbsp fat-free French-style dressing
85 g watercress

Slice the cucumber thickly, then cut each slice into quarters. Chop the tomatoes into chunks. Mix together with the beans and tuna. Drizzle with dressing, then toss together with the watercress. Serves 4.

Nicholas Culpeper the 16th century herbalist, wrote in his Herbal that the juices of watercress mixed with vinegar were good for those who were dull and lethargic, and that watercress potage (soup) was excellent for cleansing the blood in spring. The ancient Greeks believed it sharpened the wits, and the philosopher Francis Bacon (1561-1626) claimed that it could restore the bloom of youth to women (if only!). Anyway, the Romans and Angles believed in it as a cure for baldness in men. Today's herbalists say that it can cure, or help to cure, cancer. Napoleon ate watercress at almost every meal. At least it supplies us with iron and vitamin C, both important nutrients, and it goes well with fish, balancing up the solid protein and the oils.

## Fish Fillets with Dill and Cucumber
4 fillets (either salmon, sole, sea bass, cod or snapper) about 550 g/1 ¼ lb
1½ tsp lemon juice
1 clove of garlic, crushed
2 tbsp fresh dill, chopped, or 1 tsp dried
For the sauce:
150 ml/ 5 fl oz low-fat natural yoghurt or half-light sour cream
50 g/ 2 oz cucumber, finely chopped or grated
1 tbsp spring onion, chopped
freshly ground pepper

Arrange the fillets in a single layer in the grill pan. Brush with lemon juice and sprinkle with garlic and dill. Grill for 6-8 minutes or until the fish flakes easily. Meanwhile, combine the yoghurt or sour cream, cucumber, onion and pepper and spread over the fish. Grill for 2 minutes. Serves 4.

## Kedgeree
180 g/ 6 oz Patna rice
450 g/ 1 lb smoked haddock
4 eggs, hard-boiled
Curry spices: coriander, cumin, turmeric, ginger, cinnamon, chilli, or
        ready-made curry powder
seasoning
50 g/ 2 oz butter or spread
chopped parsley

Boil the rice until tender, say 15 minutes. Meanwhile poach the haddock and sieve the eggs. Cook the curry powder or spices and seasoning in butter for 3 minutes, then add the cooked, drained rice and the fish, broken up with a fork. Add half the sieved eggs, blend everything together and heat through. Place on a dish, cover with the rest of the eggs and sprinkle with the parsley.

Mrs Kate Bridges, an Edwardian cook, called kedgeree 'a man's dish'. It was brought over from India by the British army, where it was known as *khichari* and was traditionally a native vegetarian meal of lentils, rice, onions and curried eggs. Cooks in England added the smoked haddock, and kedgeree became a favourite breakfast dish. 'Serve a good breakfast,' wrote Mrs Bridges, 'and the rest of the day's dishes will be better received.' Today kedgeree is an any-time snack meal.

## Butter Bean and Fish Pie

450 g/ 1 lb plaice, skinned
100 g/ 4 oz mushrooms, quartered
450 ml/ ³/₄ pt milk
50 g/ 2 oz butter or spread
50 g/ 2 oz flour
black pepper and a pinch of sea salt
3 tbsp parsley, freshly chopped
425 g/ 15 oz can butter beans, drained
3 eggs, hard-boiled and halved
675 g/ 1¹/₂ lb mashed potato

Poach the fish and mushrooms in 300 ml/ ¹/₂ pt of the milk, seasoned. Strain the fish and mushrooms and reserve the milk. Make the white sauce by melting butter and adding flour. Cook for 1 minute. Remove from the heat and gradually stir in the milk reserved from the fish and the remaining 150 ml/¹/₄ pt. Boil to thicken, stirring all the time. Add the flaked fish, mushrooms, parsley and butter beans to the sauce mixture. Gently stir in the hard-boiled eggs. Put the whole mixture in an ovenproof dish and cover with mashed potato, dotted with butter or spread. Cook in a moderate oven until the potato is nicely browned, about 30 minutes. Serve with green vegetable or tomato: enough for 4.

## Roasted Monkfish

675 g/ 1 lb 8 oz skinned monkfish tail
4 garlic cloves, peeled
seasoning
3 tbsp olive oil
1 onion, cut into wedges
1 small aubergine, about 300 g/ 10¹/₂ oz, cut into chunks
1 red pepper, de-seeded and cut into wedges
1 yellow pepper, de-seeded and cut into wedges
1 large courgette, about 225 g/ 8 oz, cut into wedges
1 tbsp shredded fresh basil

Remove the central bone from the fish, if not already done, and make small slits down each fillet. Cut 2 garlic cloves into thin slices and insert into the fish. Put the fish on a sheet of greaseproof paper, season to taste and drizzle over 1tbsp of the oil. Bring the top edges of the paper together and completely encase the fish. Set aside. Put the remaining garlic clove and all the vegetables into a roasting tin and sprinkle with the remaining oil, turning the vegetables so that they are coated. Roast in a pre-heated oven at 200°C/400°F/gas mark 6 for 20 minutes, turning occasionally, then put the parcel of fish on top of the vegetables and cook for another 15 to 20 minutes, or until the vegetables are tender and the fish cooked. Remove the tin from the oven and open up the parcel. Cut the monkfish into thick slices. Arrange the vegetables on a serving dish, top with the fish slices and sprinkle with basil. Serve immediately.

This dish is low in carbohydrates and calories but supplies plenty of protein. Olive oil is a monounsaturated fat the remains stable at moderate temperatures and does not harm the body as some other fats may when heated.

Fish, not only the fatty type, is the healthiest source of protein. White fish, such as cod or haddock, is an excellent source of vitamin A, a protection to the heart, liver, eyes and to the skin against excess light, pollution and toxins.

**Braised Seafood with Fennel**
550 g/ 1 lb 4 oz assorted seafood such as salmon, cod, swordfish, tiger
        prawns, squid
2 tbsp olive oil
1 onion, cut into wedges
1 fennel bulb, cut into thin wedges
400 g/ 14 oz canned, chopped tomatoes or fresh equivalent, skinned
150 ml/ 5 fl oz orange juice
1 tbsp orange rind, finely grated
55 g/ 7 oz black olives, pitted
seasoning
1 tbsp flat-leaved parsley, freshly chopped
fresh salad to serve

Prepare the seafood by removing and discarding skin and bones from the fish and cutting into bite-size pieces. Peel and de-vein the prawns. Cut the squid into thin slices or rings. Wash all the fish and pat dry with kitchen paper. Heat the oil over a medium heat and add the onion and fennel. Cook, stirring occasionally, for 10 minutes or until the fish begins to soften. Add the tomatoes, orange juice and rind. Bring to the boil, reduce heat and simmer for 6-8 minutes. Add the fish, but not the prawns or squid, and simmer a further 5 minutes. Then add the remaining seafood and the olives. Cook for a further 4-5 minutes until all the seafood is tender. Season to taste and sprinkle with parsley. Serve with a fresh salad such as baby spinach leaves, watercress, chicory and orange segments.

Fennel is particularly useful in diverticular disorders since it inhibits spasm of the muscles of the digestive system and so reduces flatulence and bloating.

## Mixed Fish Kebabs

8 thin rashers of streaky bacon
8 scallops, fresh or defrosted frozen
250 g/ 9 oz monkfish, fresh or defrosted, cubed
8 whole raw prawns
olive oil

Preheat the barbecue or grill to moderate heat. Stretch each rasher of bacon with the back of a knife and wrap round the scallops. Thread the wrapped scallops, monkfish and prawns alternately on a skewer  do not squash together (if using wooden skewers, soak them in water for 20 minutes before cooking). Brush with olive oil. Pace the filled skewers on the barbecue or under the grill. Cook, turning once. Serve with couscous, barbecued/roasted vegetables or salad.

## Salmon and Cucumber Mousse

1 sachet powdered gelatine
150 ml/ 5 fl oz very hot vegetable or fish stock
418 g can Alaska red salmon with skin and bones removed
100 g/ 4 oz cucumber, peeled and chopped
3 tbsp low-fat mayonnaise
45 ml/ 3 tbsp dry white wine
150 ml/ 5 fl oz natural yoghurt
30 ml/ 2 tbsp lemon juice
2 tsp dill or parsley, finely chopped
2 egg whites
salt and freshly ground black pepper to taste
lemon or cucumber slices, fresh dill or parsley to garnish

Dissolve the gelatine by sprinkling it over very hot stock in a jug, stirring well. Leave for a minute or two until the gelatine is fully dissolved, then cool for 10-15 minutes. Flake the salmon and mix with cucumber, mayonnaise, wine, yoghurt, lemon juice and chopped herbs, or blend in a food processor. Add the cooled gelatine liquid and mix well. Whisk the egg whites until stiff, then fold through the salmon mixture. Season to taste. Pour into a serving dish and allow to set for 2 hours in the fridge. Turn out onto a serving dish and garnish with lemon or cucumber slices and fresh herbs. Serves 10-12 – a party piece.

  If you freeze it in freezer wrap when completely set you can store the mousse in the freezer for up to two months.

## Plaice with Mushroom and Yoghurt Sauce

150 ml/¼ pt vegetable stock
1 glass white wine
100 g/ 3½ oz button mushrooms, sliced
4 x 175 g/ 6 oz fillets plaice, fresh or defrosted
700 g/ 1 lb 9 oz baby spinach
250 g/ 9 oz natural yoghurt
chopped chives to garnish

Pour the vegetable stock and wine into a shallow saucepan; reduce by heating to half the volume. Add the mushrooms and simmer for 2-3 minutes. Roll the fillets up loosely and place on top of the mushrooms. Cover with a lid and gently poach. Cook the spinach and squeeze out the water. Place on warm plates and arrange the plaice fillets on top. Add the yoghurt to the stock and mushrooms, gently heat through and pour over the fish. Sprinkle with chopped chives. Serve with boiled baby potatoes, and asparagus. Serves 4.

## Pasta Salad with Salmon and Green Beans

225 g/ 8 oz small pasta shells or macaroni
60 g/ 2½ oz cottage cheese
60 g/ 2½ oz low-fat natural yoghurt
1 tbsp fresh lemon juice
100 g/ 4 oz green beans
20 g/ × oz fresh dill, coarsely chopped
2 x 73/4 oz cans salmon, drained
freshly ground pepper
lettuce

Cook the pasta until al dente (tender but firm) in a large pot of boiling water. Drain and rinse under cold water; drain again and set aside. In a food processor or with a sieve, purée the cottage cheese. Combine and mix well with yoghurt and lemon juice. In a bowl, combine the pasta, green beans, yoghurt mixture and dill. Discard the skin from the salmon and break the flesh into chunks. Add to the pasta mixture, stir gently and add pepper to taste. Line the serving plates with lettuce leaves and pile the mixture on top. Serves 8.

This dish is easy to prepare and delicious, and the good news is that it is good for you in the battle against cholesterol according to The British Heart Foundation. One type of polyunsaturated fat, the omega-3 fatty acids from fish oils, is excellent for reducing cholesterol levels and so helps prevent atherosclerosis, the furring up of the blood vessels including the coronary arteries. Omega-3 fatty acids abound in such oily fish as salmon, pilchards, sardines, herrings, trout, mackerel and fresh tuna. Canned tuna does not provide much omega-3 fatty acid, but is a useful low-fat alternative to cheese in sandwiches or salads. The Heart Foundation does not advise taking supplements of omega-3 but suggests that we should have a fish meal two or three times a week.

# Salads

Salads are the easiest, healthiest type of meal or part of a meal. No cooking is involved, and there is certain to be plenty of vitamin C and fibre in the dish.

## Classic Tuna Salad

184 g / 5 oz can tuna in water
25 g / 1 oz celery, diced
½ oz fresh dill, chopped
2 tbsp fresh parsley, chopped
2 tbsp chives or spring onions, chopped
1 tbsp low-fat mayonnaise
2 tbsp low-fat natural yoghurt
½ tsp Dijon mustard

Mash the tuna with its juices in a bowl. Add all the other ingredients and mix well. Makes 5 servings.

## Mange-tout and Red Pepper Salad

300 g / 12 oz mange-tout
2 tbsp sesame seeds
225 g / 8 oz mushrooms, sliced
1 small red pepper, cut into thin strips
For the dressing:
1 crushed clove of garlic
125 ml / 4 fl oz orange juice
3 tbsp white wine vinegar
1 tsp sugar
freshly ground pepper
2 tbsp vegetable or walnut oil

Top and string the mange-tout and blanch in boiling water for 2 minutes or until bright green. Drain and rinse under the cold tap. Dry and set aside. Cook the sesame seeds, shaking the pan often, until they are lightly browned, then set aside. To make the dressing, combine the garlic, orange juice, vinegar, sugar and black pepper in a blender or in a mixing bowl and gradually add the walnut oil. Combine the mange-tout, mushrooms and red pepper in a salad bowl and, just before serving, add the sesame seeds, pour over the dressing and toss gently. A colourful dish suitable for a buffet. Serves 8.

## Cucumber Cool

1 cucumber
¼ tsp salt
60 g/ 2½ oz sour cream or fromage frais
60 g/ 2½ oz low-fat natural yoghurt
2 tbsp chopped chives
2 tsp lemon juice
1 tbsp chopped fresh basil, or ¼ tsp dried
¼ tsp granulated sugar
freshly ground black pepper

Peel the cucumber only if tough or waxy. Slice thinly into a colander and sprinkle with salt. Toss and put aside for 30 minutes. Rinse, then pat dry. In a bowl mix the fromage frais, yoghurt, chives, lemon juice, basil and sugar. Stir in the cucumber and season with pepper. Serve in a shallow dish: enough for 6.

This is a slimming dish: 2 g fat, 33 calories and only 1 g of protein. It will require vegetable or animal protein at another meal, or combined with this.

## Danish Potato Salad

1 kg/ 2 lb potatoes
230 g/ 9 oz low-fat natural yoghurt
3 tbsp low-calorie mayonnaise
40 g/ ½ oz spring onion, finely chopped
1 tsp curry powder
1 tsp Dijon mustard
¼ tsp salt
12 g/ ½ oz dill, freshly chopped
freshly ground pepper
watercress to garnish (optional)

Wash the potatoes and cook in boiling water until tender. Drain, cool slightly. Peel only if the skins are tough. Cut into thin slices. Mix in a bowl the yoghurt, mayonnaise, onion, curry powder, mustard and salt. Add the potatoes, dill and pepper to taste, and stir. Garnish with a sprig of watercress. Makes enough for 6.

Comparison of this salad using yoghurt, low-fat mayonnaise or normal mayonnaise as dressing:
- Low-fat natural yoghurt: fat 4 g, calories 169
- Low-calorie mayonnaise: fat 16 g, calories 269
- Mayonnaise: fat 33 g, calories 420

Potato skins produce twice as much fibre as the rest of the potato.

### Family Salad from Cumbria

1 lettuce Cos, Iceberg, round, Webb or red leaf according to season
225 g/ 8 oz tomatoes, quartered
4 eggs, hard-boiled and quartered
¼ cucumber, sliced
1 stick of celery
1 carrot
100 g/ 4 oz red or white cheese, or half of each
1 box of cress

Cut up the lettuce with scissors and arrange over a serving dish, topped with tomato, eggs and cucumber. Cut the celery into small pieces and grate the carrot and cheese. Sprinkle over the salad with the cress. Serves 4.

### Summer Chicken Salad

1 grapefruit
½ melon
1 green pepper
225 g/ 8 oz cooked chicken, diced
lettuce, cucumber and watercress to garnish
For the dressing:
150 ml/ ¼ pt natural yoghurt
1 tsp lemon juice
1 tbsp finely chopped spring onions
pinch of dry mustard, salt and pepper

Chop the grapefruit flesh, scoop out balls of melon and slice the green pepper. Mix together with the chicken in a salad bowl. Mix all the dressing ingredients together, pour over the chicken mixture and toss gently. Serve on a bed of lettuce, garnished with cucumber and watercress. Sufficient for 2 or 3.

### Spinach Salad with Sesame Seed Dressing

450 g/ 1 lb spinach
50 g/ 2 oz sliced almonds

225 g / 8 oz firm strawberries, sliced
For the dressing:
1 tbsp sesame seeds
3 tbsp cider vinegar
3 tbsp vegetable or walnut oil
3 tbsp water
$\frac{1}{4}$ tsp sugar
1 tsp poppy seeds
$\frac{1}{4}$ tsp paprika
$\frac{1}{4}$ tsp Worcester sauce
1 spring onion, minced

Trim, wash and dry the spinach and tear into bite-size pieces. Set aside. Sprinkle the almonds on a baking sheet and roast until golden brown. Set aside. Meanwhile place the sesame seeds in an ungreased pan and stir over a medium heat until lightly browned. Mix thoroughly in a bowl the sesame seeds, vinegar, oil, water, sugar poppy seeds, paprika, Worcester sauce and spring onion. Just before serving, pour the dressing over the spinach and toss to coat. Add the strawberries and almonds. Toss some more. Makes 10 servings.

Wedges of mandarin oranges, grapefruit segments or sliced green apple may be used instead of strawberries.

**Cheddar Cheese and Apple Salad**
$\frac{1}{2}$ round lettuce
150 ml / 5 fl oz soured cream or natural yoghurt
3 tbsp fresh milk
1 tsp lemon juice
freshly ground pepper and pinch of salt
2 eating apples, peeled, cored and diced
225 g / 8 oz English cheddar cheese, diced
2 canned pineapple rings, drained and chopped
parsley to garnish

Wash the lettuce and shake the water off. Tear it into bite-size pieces and cover the bottom of a dish. Combine the soured cream or yoghurt with the milk, lemon juice and seasoning. Add the apples, cheese and pineapple, mix well and pile onto the lettuce. Garnish with parsley.

Pears may be used instead of apples.

Apples are as good for you as the old saying goes, 'an apple a day keeps the doctor away'. They are full of fibre and vitamin C and contain no sodium or cholesterol. They are calming to the digestion, low in calories, and chewing them cleans the teeth. They make a useful snack at any time. We have been eating apples since before 800 BC. They were originally found in Kazakhstan and quickly caught on, spreading rapidly through Asia and North Africa to Europe, wherever there was a temperate climate.

## Cottage Cheese Salad
225 g/ 8 oz back bacon, chopped
1 Cos or Webb's lettuce (crisp)
450 g/ 1 lb fresh spinach
150 ml/ ¼ pt olive oil
1 tsp dry mustard
1 tsp sugar
1 tbsp very finely grated onion
freshly ground pepper, touch of salt
4 tbsp cider or wine vinegar
225 g/ 8 oz cottage cheese

Dry-fry the bacon until crisp, then pat with absorbent kitchen paper to remove tany excess fat. Wash and drain the lettuce and spinach. Tear the leaves into bite-size pieces, discarding the stems. Mix well with the chopped bacon in a bowl. Mix the oil with the mustard, sugar, onion and seasoning. Beat in the vinegar. Pour half over the lettuce, spinach and bacon and toss well. Mix the cottage cheese with the remaining dressing and spoon into the centre of the salad greens. Serves 4.

## Chicken and Chinese Leaf Salad
1 Chinese leaf cabbage, shredded
½ onion, any colour, thinly sliced
4 handfuls of cooked chicken chunks
For the dressing:
½ clove crushed garlic
2 tsp sesame oil
1 tbsp soy sauce
juice of 2 limes or lemons
1 tsp grated ginger
1 tbsp honey
1 small minced green chilli
2 tbsp olive oil

Mix the salad ingredients together in a bowl. Combine the dressing ingredients, pour over the salad and toss well. Serves 4.

Optional additions: sliced cucumber, broccoli, green pepper, avocado, tomato or bean sprouts.

## Lee Salad
1 grapefruit
2 oranges
1 lettuce
2 apples
2 pears
juice of large lemon
$1/2$ head of celery
100 g / 4 oz grapes
50 g / 2 oz chopped walnuts
French dressing with fresh chopped mint
seasoning

Peel the grapefruit and oranges and place the segments into a bowl. Drain off any juice. Place the washed, and dried lettuce leaves in salad bowl. Wash, core and slice the apples and pears, sprinkle with lemon juice and add to grapefruit and orange segments. Add the chopped celery. Cut each grape in half and remove pips. Save a few for decoration and mix the remainder into a bowl with half the walnuts. Toss all this in the minty French dressing with some seasoning. Turn into a salad bowl and garnish with the reserved grapes and walnuts. Enough for 4-6. This recipe comes from Mrs Lee in Dumfries.

Another recipe supplying plenty of vitamins, fibre and some protein from the walnuts.

## Salade de Laitues (Lettuce Salad)
1 lettuce
1 tbsp olive oil
1 dsp of wine vinegar
$1/2$ tsp chopped tarragon
1 tsp chopped chives
$1/4$ tsp mustard
black pepper
pinch of sugar
pinch of salt
$1/2$ clove of garlic

Wash the inner leaves of a lettuce and drain in a salad basket. Mix together the oil, vinegar, tarragon, chives, mustard, black pepper and sugar. Rub the inside of a salad bowl with a pinch of salt and the garlic. Put the dry, crisp lettuce into the salad bowl and cover with the dressing. Toss with a wooden salad spoon and fork.

## Pasta Salad with Salmon and Green Beans
225 g/ 8 oz macaroni
100 g/ 4 oz green beans
60 g/ 2½ oz cottage cheese
60 g/ 2½ oz low-fat natural yoghurt
1 tbsp fresh lemon juice
20 g/ ¼ oz fresh dill, coarsely chopped
220 g/ 7 ¾ oz canned salmon, drained
freshly ground pepper
lettuce

Cook the pasta in boiling water until al dente. Rinse in cold water and drain thoroughly. Set aside. Cut the beans into 4 cm/ 1½ inch lengths and blanch in boiling water for 2 minutes. Drain and rinse in cold water. Set aside. Sieve or purée the cottage cheese and combine with the yoghurt and lemon juice. Mix together with the pasta, green beans and dill. Discard the skin from the salmon and break into chunks, then mix gently with the yoghurt mixture. Add pepper to taste. Line a serving dish with lettuce leaves and mound the salad on top. Serves 8.

## Russian Salad
1 lettuce heart or Little Gem lettuce
225 g/ 8 oz potatoes, cooked and cubed
225 g/ 8 oz carrots, cooked and cubed
100 g/ 4 oz peas, cooked
100 g/ 4 oz green beans, cooked
low-fat mayonnaise
1 egg, hard-boiled and sliced
4 gherkins, sliced

Wash and dry the lettuce leaves and arrange in a salad bowl. Put the cooked vegetables into another bowl and mix gently with the mayonnaise, just enough to coat them. Pile onto the lettuce. Add garnish and serve.

## Tropicana Salad
2 large bananas
2 medium eating apples, cored and diced
2 tbsp lemon juice

2 large oranges, peeled and sliced
150 ml/ 5 fl oz natural yoghurt
1 tsp creamed horseradish sauce

Dip the banana and apple into the lemon juice and place in a bowl. Cut the orange slices into quarters and add to the fruit. Mix any remaining lemon juice with the yoghurt and horseradish. Add the fruit and stir gently.

## Sandringham Salad
350 g/ 12 oz duck meat, cooked and shredded
2 large oranges, peeled and segmented
3 tbsp raisins
1 green pepper, seeded and sliced
175 g/ 6 oz beansprouts
175 g/ 6 oz red cabbage, shredded
French dressing as required
1 tbsp soy sauce

Place the duck, fruit and vegetables in a bowl. Mix together the French dressing and soy sauce, pour over the duck mixture and toss to coat evenly.

## Roasted Vegetable Salad
1 aubergine, about 225 g/ 8 oz
1 red pepper, de-seeded
1 orange pepper, de-seeded
1 large courgette, about 175 g/ 6 oz
1 onion
2 garlic cloves
2 tbsp olive oil
seasoning
For the dressing:
1 tbsp balsamic vinegar
2 tbsp extra virgin olive oil
1 tbsp shredded fresh basil
freshly shaved Parmesan cheese to serve

Pre-heat the oven to 200°C/400°F/gas mark 6. Cut all the vegetables into even-sized wedges, place in a roasting tin and scatter the garlic over them. In a jug mix together the balsamic vinegar and olive oil stir in the shredded fresh basil, coat the vegetables and season. Roast for 40 minutes, adding a little more oil if the mix looks dry. Sprinkle with Parmesan cheese to serve.

**Asparagus Salad with Mustard Dressing**
450 g / 1 lb asparagus
175 g / 6 oz shelled young peas, or thawed from frozen
175 g / 6 oz shelled young broad beans
juice of half a lemon – or whole small lemon
1 tbsp wholegrain mustard
4 tbsp olive oil
½ tsp clear honey
freshly ground black pepper, to taste
110 g / 4 oz rocket leaves

Clean and trim away the white ends of the asparagus. Blanch the asparagus, peas and beans for 2 minutes in boiling water, or until tender. Put the lemon juice, mustard, olive oil, honey and pepper into a screw-top jar and shake well. Toss the warm vegetables in the dressing and serve on a bed of rocket leaves. Serves 4.

**Salad Choices**
Salads are ideal for light midday meals: quick to prepare and easy on the digestion, endlessly variable and delightfully colourful. Compare, for example, these choices of light lunch meals:

Healthy:
- spinach salad with very little dressing, if any
- pasta with tomato-based sauce and Parmesan cheese
- raspberry sorbet

Less so:
- cream soup
- quiche
- jam tart

Apart from the nice, low calorie count in salad and fruit meals, they are also the healthiest for vitamins and minerals. The way the food is prepared has a big effect on how much taste and nutrition remains when it reaches your plate. Vitamins A and C and some minerals dissolve in water, so it is a good idea to use the minimum and make sure that it is boiling when you add the vegetables, or steam them in a basket or very shallow water. Sugar is also very soluble, so these precautions will help keep the delicious sweetness in vegetables such as mange-tout (related to sugar snaps).

Green leafy vegetables lose much of their valuable vitamin C, ascorbic acid, just by keeping them for a few days. Keeping fruit and vegetables in the fridge before cooking them slows the rate of vitamin loss, but while the cooking itself destroys a certain amount of loss, this is not progressive.

Salad meals may need supplementing at other meals with protein dishes.

## Salad Leaves
These can add a touch of colour and freshness, as well as vitamin C, to any meal, hot and heavy or fairy-light. No cooking comes into it.

*Rocket*: this came here with the Romans and was a frequently used herb in Elizabethan and Stuart times, either raw or cooked. It has a slightly peppery taste. It has become popular again recently and goes well with pasta. The leaves are small and ragged and make a nice garnish.

*Chinese leaves*: these are a type of cabbage with long, closely packed, pale green leaves. They are fresh-tasting and crisp when raw, but can also be steamed or stir-fried.

*Lettuces*: most salads are based on lettuce, and there is a variety to choose from. The most popular are *Cos* and *Iceberg*. Both have densely packed hearts and can be cut with a bread knife. They are particularly crisp and keep well compared with the ordinary round lettuce, which tends to have a small heart and quickly becomes limp and loses a lot of its vitamin content. The Cos is long and torpedo-shaped and the Iceberg is round. It would be sacrilege to cook either of these! There is also a red version of Cos.

*Little Gem* is a small lettuce with small, slightly crinkled leaves and no definite heart. Its size makes it convenient for one or two people and it is pleasantly crisp.

*Curly leaf* adds interest to the plate. It has loose, curly leaves which keep well in the fridge.

*Lamb's lettuce*, also called 'corn salad' or 'mache', has a mild nutty flavour. It is equally good in combination or on its own and its delicate little leaves make a decorative garnish.

*Frisee*, or curly endive, looks like a wig made of curly, lacy leaves in various shades of green, yellow and nearly white. It belongs to the chicory family and has a slightly bitter taste.

*Chicory*, also known as Belgian endive, is long and cone-shaped with yellow-tipped white leaves. It can be cooked or used in salads and its roots can be roasted and ground and used as a substitute for coffee. This was commonly done in the Second World War because of the shortages, and also for economy more recently. It is distinctly bitter.

*Radicchio* has dark pinkish leaves with crisp white ribs highly decorative, especially when they are contrasted with very green salad leaves. Radicchio has a distinctive flavour and is equally good raw, grilled or fried.

Different leaves, with contrasting flavours, colours, shapes, sizes and textures make an appetizing and truly healthy dish.

**Tricolour Salad**
125 g/ 4 oz leeks, trimmed and sliced into rings
125 g/ 4 oz red pepper, cored, de-seeded and diced
2 medium oranges, 50 g/ 8 oz of flesh, peeled and cut into quartered slices
For the dressing:
1 tbsp dill, freshly chopped
1 tbsp parsley, freshly chopped
150 ml/ ¼ pt natural low-fat yoghurt
1 tsp clear honey
freshly ground black pepper
sprig of fresh dill to garnish

Mix together the leeks, red peppers and oranges in a serving dish. Blend together the dill, parsley, yoghurt, honey and pepper and pour over the salad mix. Garnish.

# Soups

Soups are quick and easy to serve, and come in limitless varieties. They can be homemade, canned or powdered instant. Homemade soups may be fiddly to prepare, but the commercial preparations have the disadvantage of containing too much salt. Excess salt can lead to high blood pressure, stroke or heart failure. It is useful always to have some homemade soup in the freezer. If you have a liquidizer, almost any vegetables or fruit can be used to make a soup.

### Chicken and Broccoli Soup
225 g/ 8 oz broccoli florets
55 g/ 2 oz unsalted butter or olive oil spread
1 onion, chopped
225 g/ 8 oz skinless, boneless cooked chicken in thin slices
25 g/ 1 oz wholemeal flour
300 ml/ 10 fl oz milk
450 ml/ 16 oz chicken stock
55 g/ 2 oz sweetcorn
25 g/ 1 oz basmati rice

Cook the broccoli in boiling water for 3 minutes. Drain. Melt the butter, add the onion and chicken and cook for 5 minutes. Take the pan off the heat and stir in the flour, then cook for 2 minutes, stirring all the time. Stir in the milk and stock add to this the basmati rice, bring to the boil and simmer for 10 minutes. Add the broccoli and sweetcorn. Season and simmer until the rice is tender.

This is a low GI and Weight Watcher's approved dish. Broccoli is a tonic to the liver – good for detoxifying alcohol.

### Tomato and Bean Soup
1 tbsp olive oil
1 chopped onion
2 cloves of garlic (optional)
2 celery sticks, chopped
1 fresh red chilli, de-seeded and chopped
1 tbsp tomato purée
1 l / 1¾ pt vegetable stock

400 g/ 14 oz tomatoes, chopped
200 g/ 7 oz canned red kidney beans, drained
300 g/ 10 oz canned cannelini beans, drained
85 g/ 3 oz brown rice, cooked
1 tbsp basil, chopped
Parmesan cheese

Heat the oil and add the onion, garlic, celery and chilli. Cook for 3 minutes. Blend the tomato puŕe with the stock and add with the tomatoes. Bring to the boil and simmer for 10 minutes. Add the kidney, cannelini beans and seasoning and simmer for a further 10 minutes, then stir in the rice and cook for 5 minutes. Serve with a sprinkle of basil and Parmesan. This is an excellent provider of vegetable protein, soluble fibre and B vitamins.

## Mother-in-law's Mushroom Soup

A well-known brand of mushroom soup contains 4 per cent mushrooms but the rest of the ingredients include modified cornflour, dried skimmed milk, wheat flour, whey protein, salt, flavouring, vegetable oil, cream, spice extract and stabilisers. By contrast this is a very simple country recipe from Yorkshire.

250 g/ 10 oz mushrooms
300 ml/ ½ pt milk
300 ml / ½ pt chicken stock
25 g/ 1 oz plain flour
pinch of salt and pepper
50 g/ 2 oz butter

Peel and chop the mushrooms and place them in a saucepan. Stir in 250 ml/ 9fl oz of the milk and chicken stock, bring to the boil and simmer until tender. In a separate saucepan make a paste with the plain flour, a pinch of salt and pepper and 50 ml/ 2 fl oz cold milk, gently heat and transfer into the soup stirring until it thickens. Add the butter, serve with a chunk of bread.

The flavour of this soup is definitely mushroomy, and it contains antioxidants a general boost to health. The recipe lacks a variety of vegetables but any leftovers can be incorporated, or raw vegetables such as aubergine or grated carrots.

Vitamin C survives brief cooking, as do the antioxidants.

## Wayfarer's Soup

This is the essence of Nature. It sounds romantic, but is only feasible in the country.

½ bucket of fresh, young nettle leaves, stripped from the stalks
4 sticks of celery
1 onion
1 carrot
1 potato
150 ml / ¼ pt milk
pinch of salt

Wash and simmer the nettles in water for 15 minutes, then remove from the water and liquidize to a puŕe. In 600 ml/ 1 pt water simmer the roughly chopped vegetables until they are soft – about half-an-hour then liquidize. Add the nettle purée and milk, season and reheat. Serve with croutons of toast.

This is a recipe from Kent that provides iron, one of the elements we often lack. Alternatives to the nettles, and similarly beneficial, are watercress or spinach.

## Cream of Vegetable Soup
1-2 potatoes
1 leek
any other available vegetables (carrot, turnip, swede, sprout, aubergine etc.), roughly chopped
pinch of salt
300 ml/ ½ pt full-cream milk

Cover the vegetables with water, add pepper and a pinch of salt, and boil or microwave until they are just tender. Purée, and add milk to the right consistency. Reheat. Serve with hot rolls, plus cheese to increase the protein.

## Summer Fruit Soup
100 g/ 4 oz strawberries, raspberries or blackberries
or 1 large apple, pear, peach or nectarine
or 1 grapefruit or large orange
or 1 ripe banana with 100 g/ 4 oz redcurrants or blackcurrants
or 100 g/ 4 oz cherries or grapes
50 g/ 2 oz sugar
also juice and pared rind of a lemon
300 ml/ ½ pt ginger ale
fresh mint leaves or thinly sliced cucumber to garnish

Prepare the fruit of choice - that is, mash or liquidize soft fruit, peel and segment citrus, peel and chop apple or pear, or stone, peel and slice peach or nectarine. Make a syrup by simmering the sugar and lemon rind in 300 ml/ ½ pt water for 10 minutes. Strain and leave to cool. Add the lemon juice, cooled syrup and ginger ale to the chosen fruit. Serve with ice cubes and mint or cucumber.

This refreshing soup is full of vitamin C, antioxidants and fibre. Essential fats and protein will be needed at other meals in the day.

## Grilled Vegetable Soup
2 onions, halved but not peeled
1-3 cloves of garlic, according to taste
4 ripe tomatoes
2 aubergines, halved lengthways
2 red peppers, halved and de-seeded
sprigs of thyme
1 bay leaf if available
1 tbsp olive oil
1 l/ 1¾ pt vegetable stock
juice of freshly-squeezed lemon
black pepper
handful of torn basil leaves

Put the onions, garlic, tomatoes, aubergines and peppers under the grill for 10 minutes, or until softened and beginning to char. Cool slightly and peel the onion, garlic and tomatoes. Chop coarsely. Heat the thyme and bay leaf gently in the olive oil for 2 minutes, then add the vegetables and stock. Bring to the boil, cover and simmer for 20 minutes or microwave for 5 minutes, then leave to cool. Remove the bay leaf. Process the soup briefly in the liquidizer, so that it retains some of its texture. Return the soup to the pan, add the lemon juice and pepper to season, and reheat. Serve garnished with basil leaves.

This soup has a wonderful flavour and is packed with vitamins A, C and E and vegetable protein.

## Leek and Sweetcorn Soup
25 g/ 1 oz butter or vegetable oil spread
450 g/ 1 lb leeks, sliced
2 celery sticks, sliced
1 onion, sliced
198 g/ 7 oz can sweetcorn, drained
450 ml/¾ pt vegetable stock
50 g/ 2 oz grated cheese

25 g/ 1 oz cornflour
450 ml/ ¾ pt milk

Cook the butter, leeks, celery and onion until soft. Add the sweetcorn and stock, bring to the boil, cover and simmer for 15 minutes. Remove from the heat and stir in half the cheese. Serve topped with the rest of the cheese.

This soup has a good balance of the essential nutrients: carbohydrate, essential fats and protein, as well as fibre and vitamins.

**Savoy Cabbage Soup**
4 rashers streaky bacon, finely diced
1 onion, minced
1 head Savoy cabbage, cut into 1½-inch cubes
generous pinch of dried thyme
1.5 l/ 2½ pt hot chicken or vegetable stock
200 ml natural yoghurt
seasoning to taste
100 g smoked trout, mackerel or salmon, shredded

Cook the bacon in a large stockpot on a medium heat for 4 minutes, until crisp. Add the onion and cook for another 5 minutes or until tender, stirring. Add the cabbage and thyme, stir for 3 minutes, then add stock and bring to the boil. Reduce the heat, simmer for about 20 minutes, add the yoghurt and simmer for 5 minutes more. Season to taste. Spoon into bowls and top with shredded, smoked fish. Serves 4-6.

Cabbage sounds commonplace and unromantic, but it has a long and distinguished history. In Ancient Greece it was said to have been made from the sweat of Zeus, the top god, while the Romans thought it made people live longer. The Ancient Egyptians valued it even more as a way of drinking heavily without ill effects. Russian princes made gifts or paid tributes not only with jewels and racehorses, but also plots of land planted with *kopusta* – cabbage. Cabbages have featured on the British menu since around 6000 BC and became popular when the Savoy was introduced from Italy in the 16th century. Cabbages are a valuable source of fibre and vitamin C, and Savoys contain five times as much beta-carotene as the others.

**Soups from Other Countries**

Every land has its own characteristic soup. All of them are suitable for those with diverticulitis, particularly because of their fibre content and wide variety of ingredients.

## Austria

**Hot Apple Soup** *(Apfelsuppe)*
459 g/ 1 lb cooking apples
grated rind of 1 lemon
small glass of white wine (optional)
2 ¼ pt water
1 – 2 tbsps / 25 g sugar
225 g/ 8 oz currants
225 g/ 8 oz sultanas
25 g/ 1 oz butter
1 tbsp/ 1 oz cornflour

Cut up the apples, including the skin and core, grate the lemon rind over them and cook in the wine or a little water until they are soft. Liquidize and add water, sugar, currants and sultanas. Simmer for 30 minutes. Melt the butter and stir into the apple mixture together with the cornflour. Simmer for another 10 minutes.

While potato soup seems natural, apple soup sounds unusual. In fact potatoes are known as 'earth apples' in some languages, for instance *pommes de terre* in French or *aardappels* in Dutch. The name 'potato' comes from the Spanish *batata*. It was the Spaniards who introduced potatoes to Europe from South America – and they have certainly taken root.

## Bulgaria

**Cabbage and Bacon Soup** *(Zeleva Chorba sas Beton)*
1 small cabbage
1 onion, chopped
175 g/ 6 oz bacon, diced
30 ml/ 2 tbsp vegetable oil
flour to thicken
black pepper
caraway seeds
1 egg, beaten
60 ml/ 4 tbsp sour milk

Slice the cabbage finely and cook in sufficient water. Meanwhile heat the chopped onion and diced bacon in oil until they are soft, then stir in the flour. Pour over the cabbage. Add the pepper, caraway seeds, well-beaten egg and sour milk. Mix and heat without boiling.

## Holland Cookery
Farmer's Soup
3 potatoes
3 rashers of bacon
55 g/ 2 oz dried mushrooms or 100 g fresh mushrooms
$1\frac{1}{2}$ l/ 3 pt stock
2 bay leaves
225 g/ 8 oz sauerkraut
150 ml/ 5 fl oz full-cream milk
15 ml/ 1 tbsp flour

Cut the potatoes, bacon and mushrooms into small pieces, add to the stock with the bay leaves and cook for 20 minutes. Liquidize or sieve and add the sauerkraut, milk and flour to thicken. Reheat.

## France

## French Onion Soup (*Soupe à l'Oignon*)
350 g/ 12 oz onions, thinly sliced
40 g/ $1\frac{1}{2}$ oz butter or olive oil spread
900 ml/ $1\frac{1}{2}$ pt beef stock (cube)
pinch of salt and freshly ground pepper
4 slices of French bread, 2.5 cm/ 1-inch thick
50 g/ 2 oz grated Cheddar cheese

Gently fry the onions in butter or spread until golden. Add the stock, season and bring to the boil, then simmer for 45 minutes. You may cover and microwave for 15 minutes if you prefer. In individual dishes, float the bread on top of the soup, sprinkle with cheese and brown under the grill. Serves 4.

## Germany

## Egg Barley Soup (*Eiergerstensuppe*)
1 whole egg
1 egg yolk
flour to thicken
$1\frac{1}{2}$ pt clear beef stock
1 dsp chives, chopped
1 dsp dry horseradish, grated
parsley, finely chopped

Mix the beaten egg, egg yolk and flour to make a stiff ball. Leave for 1 hour, then grate on a coarse grater. Spread on a dish and leave to dry. Bring the stock to the boil, sprinkle over the chives and horseradish and cook for 5 minutes. Garnish with parsley.

## Hungary

**Fish Goulash Soup** *(Halaszli)*
450 g/ 1 lb haddock or other fish
850ml /1½ pt water
2 tsp paprika
2 onions, chopped
1 green pepper, de-seeded and cut into strips
1 tbsp butter or vegetable oil
salt to taste (minimum)

Fillet the fish and put the bones in a saucepan with water, paprika and chopped onions. Cover and simmer for 30 minutes. Cut the fish into small pieces and, together with the chopped pepper, add to the strained fish stock. Simmer until the fish is tender. Add salt to taste only if necessary. Serve with butter or oil.

## Poland

**Dried Mushroom Soup** *(Zupa Grzybowa)*
50 g/ 2 oz dried mushrooms
850ml / 1½ pt stock
seasoning to taste, minimum salt
25 g/ 1 oz butter or oil
25 g/ 1 oz flour
45 ml/ 3 tbsp soured cream

Blanch the mushrooms and simmer in seasoned stock. Heat the butter and flour for 1 minute, then gradually add the stock and mushrooms. Stir in the soured cream.

## Russia

**Georgian Soup** *(Kharcho)*
450 g/ 1 lb mutton
1.5 l/ 3 pt water
seasoning
1 onion

1 tbsp butter
1 tbsp flour
225 g/ 8 oz tomatoes
2 cloves of garlic
225 g/ 8 oz sour plums
225 g/ 8 oz rice
sprig of dill

Cut the meat into pieces, allowing 3 for each person Simmer in water with seasoning for $1^1/_2$ hours, or microwave until tender. Chop the onion finely and fry in butter. Blend in the flour and mix with the skinned, quartered tomatoes. Add to the meat stock together with the crushed garlic, plums and rice. Simmer for 20 minutes. Serve into individual plates and sprinkle with chopped dill. Serves 4.

## Borscht
1 onion, chopped
450 g/ 1 lb raw beetroot, peeled and chopped
2 celery sticks, chopped
§ red pepper, chopped
115 g/ 4 oz mushrooms, chopped
1 large cooking apple, chopped
25 g / 1 oz butter
30 ml/ 2 tbsp sunflower oil
2 l/ $3^1/_2$ pt stock or water
5 ml/ 1 tsp cumin seeds
pinch of dried thyme
1 large bay leaf
fresh lemon juice
salt and freshly ground black pepper
For the garnish:
150 ml/ $^1/_4$ pt soured cream
few sprigs of fresh dill

Place the chopped vegetables and apple in a large saucepan with butter, oil and 45 ml/ 3 tbsp of the stock or water. Cover and cook gently for about 15 minutes, shaking the pan occasionally. Stir in the cumin seeds and cook for 1 minute, then add the remaining stock or water, thyme, bay leaf, lemon juice and seasoning to taste. Bring the mixture to the boil, then cover and turn down the heat to a gentle simmer. Cook for about 30 minutes. Strain the vegetables and reserve the liquid. Process the vegetables in a processor or blender until smooth and creamy. Return the vegetables to the pan, add the reserved stock and reheat. Check the seasoning. Divide into 6 individual serving bowls. Garnish with swirls of soured cream topped with sprigs of fresh dill.

This is a classic Russian soup, with a wonderful rich colour and flavour to match. The flavour matures if made the day before. An excellent winter warmer.

## Scandinavia

### Cauliflower Soup *(Blomkal Suppe)*
900g / 2 lb cauliflower
600 ml/ 1 pt water
600 ml/ 1 pt stock
seasoning, minimal salt
2 egg yolks
45 ml/ 3 tbsp chopped parsley

Break the cauliflower into sections, discarding the tough stalk. Simmer in the water until soft. Beat the cauliflower with a whisk, add the stock, bring to the boil and season to taste. Stir in the beaten egg yolks and parsley.

## Spain

### Castilian Garlic Soup *(Sopa de Ajo a la Castellano)*
4 slices white bread
2 cloves of garlic
30 ml/ 2 tbsp olive oil
seasoning
850ml / 1½ pt water

Cut the crusts off the bread. Pound the garlic and fry in oil. When golden, add the bread and fry lightly, season and add the cold water. Bring to the boil and simmer for 10 minutes.

This soup is made in almost every Spanish home. It tastes good but contains little nourishment, so there needs to be something more substantial in the other meals.

## Japan

### Japanese Crushed Tofu Soup
150 g/ 5 oz fresh tofu, weighed without water
2 dried shiitake mushrooms

50 g/2 oz gobo
5 ml/1 tsp rice vinegar
½ black or white konnyaku (about 115 g/4 oz)
30 ml/2 tbsp sesame oil
115 g/4 oz mooli, finely sliced
50 g/2 oz carrot, finely sliced
750 ml/1¼ pt kombu and bonito stock, or instant dashi
pinch of salt
30 ml/2 tbsp sake or dry white wine
7.5 ml/1½ tsp mirin
45 ml/3 tbsp white or red miso paste
dash of soy sauce
6 mange-tout, trimmed, boiled and finely sliced to garnish

Crush the tofu roughly by hand until it resembles lumpy scrambled egg in texture – do not crush it too finely. Wrap in a clean tea towel and put it in a sieve, then pour over plenty of boiling water. Leave the tofu to drain thoroughly for 10 minutes. Soak the dried shiitake mushrooms in tepid water for 20 minutes, then drain. Remove the stems and cut the caps into 4-6 pieces. Use a vegetable brush to rub the skin off the gobo and slice into thin shavings. Soak the shavings for 5 minutes in plenty of cold water with the vinegar added to remove any bitter taste. Drain. Put the konnyaku in a small saucepan and cover with water. Bring to the boil, then drain and cool. Tear the konnyaku into 2 cm/ ¾-inch lumps – do not use a knife, as smooth cuts will prevent it from absorbing the flavour. Heat the sesame oil in a deep pan, add all the shiitake mushrooms, gobo, mooli, carrot and konnyaku. Stir-fry for 1 minute, then add the tofu and stir well. Pour in the stock or dashi and add the salt, sake or wine, and mirin. Bring to the boil. Skim the broth and simmer it for 5 minutes. In a small bowl, dissolve the miso paste in a little of the soup, then return it to the pan. Simmer the soup gently for 10 minutes, until the vegetables are soft. Add the soy sauce, then remove from the heat. Serve immediately in 4 bowls, garnished with the mange-tout.

Cooking, or attempting to cook, this soup might be fun to try once as an example of a Japanese dish, but you would need plenty of leisure time to do it often. It would be vital to obtain and line up all the ingredients, pans, sieve, vegetable brush, clean tea towel and a good helping of patience before you begin!

# Main Meals

The main meal of the day is usually either at midday or in the evening, although breakfast can run a close second. The important ingredient of the main meal is protein: meat, fish, dairy products including eggs, and some vegetables. Protein is essential for growth and repair, and is also used as fuel when there is a shortage of carbohydrate. However, there is a high fat content in many meats, which may lead to an unhealthily high cholesterol level. For example, some cafés and restaurants advertise an 'all-day breakfast' which is likely to provide bacon, eggs and sausages – plenty of protein but also high in fat.

### High-fat meats (30-40 per cent of weight raw):

- duck, especially the skin
- streaky and back bacon
- best end of lamb and loin
- belly of pork

### Moderately high-fat meats (20-30 per cent of weight raw):
- loin and leg of pork
- scrag, middle neck and shoulder of lamb
- goose
- sirloin steak
- forerib of beef

### Moderately fat meats (10-20 per cent of weight raw):
- leg of lamb and lamb's liver
- chicken, with skin
- beef mince
- rump steak
- topside of beef
- stewing steak
- ox tongue

### Low-fat meats (5-10 per cent of weight raw)
- pheasant
- ox liver

- partridge
- calves' liver
- turkey, including skin
- pig's liver
- chicken liver

**Very low fat meats (less than 5 per cent of weight raw)**
- duck, without skin
- chicken, without skin
- turkey, without skin
- rabbit
- lamb's kidney
- pig's kidney
- ox kidney
- clean veal

## Comparison of High-Fat and Low-Fat Ham Dinner

### Dinner 1: 29 per cent of calories from fat

| | | |
|---|---|---|
| Cauliflower and ham gratin | 10 g fat | 219 calories |
| Green beans | 0.1 g fat | 17 calories |
| Sliced tomatoes | 0.1 g fat | 2 calories |
| Wholemeal roll | 1.0 g fat | 90 calories |
| Margarine 1 tsp | 3.6 g fat | 34 calories |
| Milk, skimmed, ½ pt | 0 g fat | 90 calories |
| Total | 15 g fat | 461 calories |

### Dinner 2: 47 per cent of calories from fat

| | | |
|---|---|---|
| Ham steak | 8.7 g fa | 187 calories |
| Cauliflower | 0.1 g fat | 14 calories |
| Cheese sauce | 9.9 g fat | 126 calories |
| Wholemeal roll | 0.1 g fat | 90 calories |
| Butter 1 tsp | 3.6 g fat | 34 calories |
| Whole milk, ½ pt | 9 g fat | 159 calories |
| Total | 32.4 g fat | 627 calories |

## Recipes

**Barbecued Lemon Chicken**
4 skinless, boneless chicken breasts
juice of 1 lemon
2 tbsp olive oil

1 clove of garlic, crushed
½ tsp dried oregano
pinch of cayenne pepper

Arrange the chicken in a single layer in a shallow dish. In a small dish combine the lemon juice, oil, garlic, oregano and cayenne, mixing well. Pour over the chicken, coating both sides, cover and stand at room temperature for 20 minutes. On a preheated, greased grill or over barbecue coals, cook the chicken for 4-5 minutes on each side, until the flesh is no longer pink. Serves 4.

## Tuna Steaks with Pesto Coating
2 slices of wholemeal bread, crumbled
2 tsp pesto
2 x 175 g/ 6 oz tuna steaks, fresh or defrosted
salad leaves and tomato to garnish

Preheat the grill or barbecue to moderate temperature. Mix the breadcrumbs and pesto together. Wipe the tuna and firmly press the mixture onto the fish. Cook gently, turning once and checking with a fork – there should be no resistance. Take care not to overcook this beautiful fish. Serve garnished with the salad.
   A healthy meal low in fat and a low glycaemic index.

## Fruity Lamb Stew
700 g/ 1½ lb boneless leg of lamb, trimmed and cubed
1 medium onion, chopped
½ tsp ground ginger
½ tsp ground coriander
½ tsp ground cinnamon
900 ml/1½ pt stock
50 g/ 2 oz no-soak dried prunes, stoned and halved
50 g/ 2 oz no-soak dried apricots, halved
cooked rice to serve

Put the lamb, onion, spices and stock in a saucepan. Bring to the boil, cover and simmer for 1¼ hours. Add the fruit and bring back to the boil. Simmer for 15 minutes. Serve with cooked rice. Alternatively, this dish can be microwaved in 40 minutes.

## Summer Rice Salad with Cheshire Cheese
200 g/ 7 oz long grain and wild rice

250 g/ 9 oz Cheshire cheese
1 piece (10 cm/ 4 in) cucumber
175 g/ 6 oz cherry tomatoes, halved
3 spring onions, thinly sliced
small handful of mint
For the dressing:
grated zest and juice of 1 small orange
grated zest and juice of 1 lemon
3 tbsp extra virgin olive oil
freshly ground black pepper to taste, pinch of salt

Cook the rice in boiling salted water for 15-18 minutes, until just tender. Drain, rinse in cold water, and drain again thoroughly. In a bowl whisk together the dressing ingredients and season to taste. Add the dressing to the rice and mix. Break the Cheshire cheese into small pieces and add to the rice. Quarter the cucumber lengthways, cut out the seeds and dice. Add to the rice with the tomatoes and spring onions. Shred the mint leaves and fold into the salad. Serve immediately.

Cheshire is our oldest named cheese. It can be used hot or cold, but when cold is best eaten at room temperature.

**Quick 'n' Easy Fish Pie**
 250 g/ 9 oz white fish (coley, cod, haddock or bass), fresh or defrosted,
       skinned, boned and cubed
250 g/ 9 oz smoked fish, cubed
1 small can of sweetcorn, drained, or prawns, button mushrooms or peas
2 tbsp chopped parsley
1 x 200 ml tub of low-fat crème fraîche
2 packs long-life 'breakfast brunch' potato or mashed potato
broccoli or green salad

Preheat the oven to 200°C/400°F/gas mark 6. In an ovenproof dish, mix the two types of fish together with the sweetcorn (or prawns, button mushrooms or peas instead of sweetcorn if preferred). Stir the parsley into the creme fraîche and pour over the fish. Spread the potato over the top and cook for 25-30 minutes. Serve with broccoli or green salad. Serves 4.

**Beef and Bean Hot Pot**
2 tbsp olive oil
8 shallots, peeled
2 celery sticks, chopped
175 g/ 6 oz carrots, cut into chunks

550 g/ 1lb 4 oz braising steak, trimmed of fat and diced
1 tbsp plain wholemeal flour
1 tbsp tomato purée
600 ml/ 1 pt beef stock
55 g/ 2 oz pearl barley, rinsed
seasoning
550 g/ 1 lb 4 oz sweet potatoes, peeled and sliced
1 tbsp chopped fresh parsley

Preheat the oven to 180°C/350°F/gas mark 4. Heat half the oil in a large saucepan over a medium heat. Add the shallots, celery and carrots and cook for 2 minutes, stirring frequently. Add the steak and cook for 2-3 minutes, stirring non-stop until the meat is sealed all over. Sprinkle in the flour, stir and cook for 2 minutes. Blend the tomato purée with a little stock and stir into the saucepan, then stir in the remaining stock and the pearl barley. Bring to the boil, stirring constantly, then reduce the heat and simmer for 5 minutes. Season to taste and transfer to an ovenproof casserole dish. Arrange the sweet potato slices on top and brush with the rest of the oil. Bake for 2-2½ hours or until the meat and vegetables are tender, taking the lid off for the last 20 minutes to crisp the top. Sprinkle with parsley.

Celery contains a chemical, apigenin, that relaxes the blood vessels and reduces the blood pressure. High blood pressure often occurs at the same age as diverticulitis.

## Haynes Landrace au Gratin
1 kg/ 2 lb bacon joint, home-produced if possible
4 shallots
450 g/ 1 lb baby carrots
450 g/ 1 lb French beans, cut into 2.5 cm/ 1-inch lengths
450 g/ 1 lb fresh peas, shelled
4 baby courgettes
4 eggs, hard-boiled
For the sauce:
50 g/ 2 oz butter
50 g/ 2 oz flour
300 ml/ ½ pt milk
100 g/ 4 oz grated Cheddar cheese
1 twist ground black pepper
To garnish:
25 g/ 1 oz grated Cheddar cheese
4 small tomatoes, sliced
sprigs of parsley

Soak the bacon joint in water for about 4 hours, then just cover with fresh water and boil for 1¼-1½ hours, adding the shallots and carrots for the last 20 minutes. Remove the vegetables and allow the bacon to cool, reserving the stock. Lightly boil the French beans and peas, slice the courgettes, halve the eggs, dice the cold bacon and arrange in layers in an ovenproof dish. Melt the butter, stir in the flour and then the milk to make a sauce. Add the cheese, pepper and sufficient bacon stock to make a pourable consistency. Pour over the vegetable mixture and sprinkle with the remainder of the grated cheese. Bake in a moderate oven until golden, about 35 minutes. Garnish with the tomatoes and parsley and serve with buttered broad beans and, if available, new potatoes.

This recipe comes from Lincolnshire. It has good variety of vegetables, but the other meals of the day should be low in fat for a healthy balance.

### Chicken, Fresh Herb and Tomato Ring

1 sachet of powdered gelatine
300 ml/ 10 fl oz very hot chicken stock
5 tbsp low-fat mayonnaise
225 g/ 8 oz plain fromage frais
30 ml/ 2 tbsp dry white wine (optional)
350 g/ 12 oz cooked, chopped chicken
2 tbsp chopped, fresh mixed herbs, such as tarragon, parsley, chives,
    marjoram
3 tomatoes, skinned and chopped
2 egg whites
freshly-ground black pepper
pinch of salt
5 cm/ 2-inch piece of cucumber
2 tomatoes, sliced
½ green or red pepper, de-seeded and chopped
3 spring onions, finely chopped
baby spinach leaves or watercress
3 tbsp low-fat vinaigrette dressing
fresh herbs to garnish

Dissolve the gelatine by sprinkling it onto very hot (not boiling) chicken stock. Stand for 2-3 minutes, stirring occasionally to produce a clear liquid. Cool for 10-15 minutes. In a large bowl mix together the mayonnaise, fromage frais, wine, chicken, herbs and tomatoes. Pour in the cooled gelatine liquid, mixing thoroughly. Whisk the egg whites until stiff, then fold into the mixture with a metal spoon. Season and pour into a 1 l/ 1¾ pt ring mould. Refrigerate until set, about 2 hours. Turn out onto a serving plate when completely set. Mix together the cucumber, tomatoes, pepper, spring onions, spinach or watercress and the vinaigrette dressing. Season to taste, then spoon into the centre of the ring. Garnish with fresh herbs. Serves 6-8.

## Ploughman's Pie
450 g/ 1 lb shortcrust pastry (to line and cover a 1l/1¼ pt pie dish using wholewheat or 50/50 wholewheat and white plain flour)
450 g/ 1 lb mutton or lamb, cooked and sliced
100 g/ 4 oz stringless runner beans, boiled for 2 minutes
2 medium cooking apples, peeled, cored, chopped and tossed in brown sugar, cinnamon and nutmeg
50 g/ 2 oz whole wheat, boiled or steamed until tender
seasoning
1 tbsp milk

Line a pie dish with shortcrust pastry keeping to one side enough to make the lid. Combine the ingredients except the milk and place in the pastry-lined pie dish, brush the edges of the pastry with milk, cover with the pastry lid. Make a small hole in the pastry lid for steam to escape and brush with milk. Decorate with scraps of pastry. Bake for 40 minutes or until golden brown at 200°C/400°F/gas mark 6. Serve cold for lunch with brown bread and tomatoes, or hot in the evening with potatoes and baby turnips.
    The other meals of the day must go easy on the calories.

## Tuna and Tortellini
300 g/ 12 oz tortellini or other pasta
150 g/ 6 oz frozen peas (fresh if available)
§ red pepper, diced
60 g/ 2½ oz red onion, chopped
1 can (184 g/ 6½ oz) tuna in water, drained
1 can (398 g/ 14 oz) artichokes, drained and quartered (optional)
20 g/ ¾ oz chopped fresh parsley
12 g/ ½ oz chopped fresh basil, or 2 tsp dried
For the dressing:
1 clove garlic, minced
1 tsp Dijon mustard
3 tbsp lemon juice or white wine vinegar
4 tbsp orange juice
3 tbsp olive oil
60 g/ 2½ oz low-fat natural yoghurt

½ oz finely chopped fresh basil
seasoning

Cook the tortellini in plenty of boiling water until al dente. Drain, rinse under cold water and drain again. Thaw peas under cold water. In a salad bowl, combine the pasta, peas, red pepper, onion, tuna, artichokes, parsley and basil. Toss lightly to mix. In a blender or bowl combine the garlic, mustard, lemon and orange juice, drizzling in the oil while mixing. Add the yoghurt, basil and seasoning. Pour over the salad and toss well. Cover to refrigerate – it will keep for 2 days. Serves 8.

Peas, whether fresh, frozen or canned, are an excellent source of fibre, iron, niacin and vitamin C. Grated carrot enhances the nutritonal value and flavour of the peas.

## Meatless Main Courses

Protein is an essential part of our nourishment. For those suffering from diverticulitis or at risk of it, it is particularly important to obtain more protein from vegetable sources and less from meat and other animal foods such as cheese, fish, eggs and dairy products. Vegetable protein is found in vegetables, legumes (beans, peas and lentils), nuts, seeds and grain. It also provides some vitamins and minerals, and is higher in fibre but lower in saturated fats than animal protein. Both of these are beneficial, but there is one snag: protein consists of 22 amino-acids, of which 13 can be produced in the body, leaving 9 so-called essential amino-acids which must be provided by our food. Animal foods all contain a full set of amino-acids, but vegetable foods do not. This means that, for adequate nourishment, you need to have some animal food in combination with plant foods, and preferably more than one type of the latter.

We tend, instinctively, to choose such combinations, for instance fish and chips – animal and plant. A big bag of chips does not make up for a lack of fish. Other 'good companions' are grain and a dairy product, such as bread and cheese or cornflakes and milk. Low-fat dairy products are often used to supplement plant foods, for instance mozzarella cheese topping with three-bean casserole, or skimmed milk in vegetable soup. Legumes with grains, such as baked beans on wholemeal toast, or legumes and nuts, as in a salad with chick peas and walnuts, provide almost all the amino-acids you need.

People who choose meatless meals from vegetarian principles often supplement their meals with eggs or cheese, both animal foods. These contain saturated fats, but they are only harmful if you frequently eat, high-fat cheeses like Cheddar and the cream cheeses, and eggs more than twice a week.

### Barley, Green Pepper and Tomato Casserole
225 g/ 8 oz pearl barley
750 ml/ 1¼ pt hot vegetable stock or water
2 onions, chopped
1 green pepper, chopped
2 large tomatoes, cut into chunks
1 tsp dried oregano
pinch of salt
freshly ground pepper
225 g/ 8 oz Cheddar cheese, grated

Combine the barley, stock, onions, green pepper, tomatoes, oregano, salt and pepper to taste in a baking dish. Stir. Cover and bake at 180°C/ 350°F/gas mark 4 for 45 minutes. Stir in the cheese and bake uncovered for a further 25 minutes or until the barley is tender and most of the liquid absorbed. Serves 6.

### Vegetable Lasagne
1 tbsp olive oil
1 small onion, chopped
3 cloves of garlic, crushed
1 carrot, chopped
1 stick of celery, chopped
150 g/ 6 oz mushrooms, sliced
1 can (540 g/ 19 oz) tomatoes
3 tbsp tomato purée
6 tbsp water
1 tsp dried basil
1 tsp dried oregano
freshly ground pepper
pinch of salt
450 g/ 1 lb small broccoli florets
9 lasagne sheets
250 g/ 10 oz cottage cheese
300 g/ 12 oz low-fat mozzarella cheese, grated
25 g/ 1 oz Parmesan cheese

In a large saucepan heat the oil gently, add the onion and cook until tender. Stir in the garlic, carrot, celery and mushrooms and cook for 5 minutes, stirring frequently. Add the tomatoes, breaking up with a fork. Stir in the tomato purée, basil and oregano, season to taste. Simmer, uncovered, until slightly thickened, about 10 minutes. Allow to cool and then stir in the broccoli. Cook the lasagne sheets in boiling water until al dente (firm but tender), drain and rinse in cold water. Over the bottom of a lightly greased baking dish arrange 3 of the sheets. Spread with half of the vegetable mixture, then half of the cottage cheese. Sprinkle with one-third of the mozzarella cheese. Repeat the layers once more. Arrange the remaining lasagne sheets over the top and sprinkle with the rest of the mozzarella and Parmesan. Bake at 180°C/350°F/gas mark 4 until hot and bubbly, about 35-45 minutes. Serves 8.

This lasagne will keep for several days in the fridge and any left over can be used for a pasta salad or reheated for a light meal. It provides fibre and iron as well as vitamins A and C, and is an excellent source of niacin and calcium. It makes a substantial meatless meal.

### Egg and Tomato Boats
4 large eggs, hard-boiled
4 large tomatoes
100 g/4 oz Cheddar cheese, cubed
2 tsp chives, chopped
2 tsp parsley, chopped
1 tbsp low-fat mayonnaise
lettuce leaves
¾ cucumber, sliced
2 tbsp red Leicester cheese, grated

Cut the eggs and tomatoes in half. Scoop out the tomato centres and egg yolks. Mix to a pulp and add the Cheddar, chives, parsley and mayonnaise. Spoon the mixture into the tomatoes and egg whites. Arrange on a bed of lettuce with the sliced cucumber and top with the grated red cheese. Serves 4.

A quick, light, meatless meal that is even better with chopped ham instead of Cheddar cheese. Eggs and cheese are the obvious sources of protein if meat and fish are to be avoided. Both of these contain a good deal of saturated fat and should not be eaten more than three times a week if meat is also in the diet.

### Winter Vegetables with Cheese
2 tbsp vegetable oil
350 g/12 oz yellow turnip, cut into thin strips
125 ml/4 fl oz water
1 red pepper, cut into thin strips
100 g/4 oz onion, thinly sliced

300 g/ 12 oz courgettes, thinly sliced
75 g/ 3 oz mushrooms, sliced
4 medium tomatoes, cut in chunks
½ tsp dried oregano
freshly ground pepper, trace of salt
1 tbsp Parmesan cheese, grated
150 g/ 6 oz low-fat mozzarella cheese, grated

Heat the oil over medium heat. Add the turnip, cover and cook for 10 minutes or until tender. Stir occasionally and add a little water if necessary. Add the red pepper and onions and cook, stirring, for 2 minutes. Add the courgettes and mushrooms and cook, stirring, for 3 minutes. Add the tomatoes and cook on, high heat, stirring occasionally, for 5-10 minutes or until excess moisture has evaporated. Stir in the oregano and season to taste. Spoon the vegetable mixture into a shallow, heatproof baking dish. Sprinkle evenly with the Parmesan and mozzarella cheeses. Grill for 3-5 minutes, until the cheese is melted and slightly browned. Serves 8.

This dish is good for fibre, vitamin A, niacin and calcium and an excellent supplier of vitamin C. Keep in the fridge, covered, and reheat when required: 3-4 minutes in the microwave on high.

# Special Diets

## Vegetarian

Vegetarians often claim that their diet is healthier than other people's: it depends on the degree of vegetarianism. There are five grades; Grades 1 and 2 provide all you need for perfect health, whilst grades 4 and 5 lead to nutritional deficiencies:

1   Avoidance of particular animal proteins, for instance horse meat, pork and bacon, or brain.
2   Cutting out red meat and poultry, but eating fish, eggs, milk and dairy products.
3   No meat, poultry or fish, but eating eggs and dairy foods: lacto-ovo-vegetarian.
4   Avoidance of all animal products: vegan.
5   Nothing but fruit: fruitarian.

The vegan diet causes a shortage of vitamin B12, which in turn leads to a form of anaemia. It is particularly dangerous for babies exclusively breast-fed by a vegan mother. The baby is likely to suffer permanently impaired mental, social and muscular development.

A fruitarian diet is incompatible with survival and leads to a shortage of protein and even such basics as salt.

## Weight Loss

Certain slimming diets are harmful and should be avoided:

1   Liquid Protein (Prolinn): combined with fasting, this has caused at least 60 deaths from irregular heart action
2   Zen Macrobiotic: 10 levels leading up to 100 per cent cereal and very little fluid. It causes kidney damage, scurvy, anaemia and shortage of calcium. Sometimes lethal.
3   The Atkins Diet: this involves a drastic reduction in carbohydrates, causing a high level of fats in the blood. There is weight loss but at the risk of high blood pressure and heart problems. Dr Atkins himself became overweight and died.

4    The Beverley Hills Diet: this starts with 10 days on fruit only, then small amounts of salad, bread and meat are added. It is condemned by the American Medical Association.

## The Polymeal

This medical nutritional breakthrough confirms what many ordinary people have always felt – that what we eat has a major effect on our health, in particular on the risk of the top killer, heart and artery disease, and length of life.

The Polymeal has superseded the Polypill, a mix of vitamins and other food essentials in pill form. The Polymeal, by contrast, consists of real food and is more natural, palatable and safer. Its ingredients can be combined and eaten at one sitting or taken separately at different times. It is recommended that it should be taken on a daily basis by age 50, in conjunction with an active, frugal lifestyle. There are seven key ingredients:

- dark chocolate
- wine
- fish, especially fatty, 2 – 4 times a week: not fried
- fruit and vegetables
- nuts
- garlic
- tea.

It takes care to provide the recommended daily portions of nuts and dark chocolate: 68 g and 100 g respectively.

Other healthy items include oat bran, cereals, soya oil and beans, chickpeas, tomatoes, olive oil, echium oil, egg yolk, watercress and apples: 'An apple a day keeps the doctor away,' as our grandmothers said. In fact, it protects the lining of the stomach and gut from damage. Filter or instant coffee is kinder to the stomach and nerves than the pure or decaffeinated types, and it is helpful to avoid getting depressed.

Driving and other activities requiring concentration should be postponed after a polymeal, and garlic is better avoided before social engagements for the sake of the other people  unless they have eaten it too! The Polymeal seems to enhance the pungency of both breath and body odour from garlic.

The weekly running cost of this diet in 2007 was approximately £21.60: wine £3.50; fruit and vegetables £6.23; almonds £2.80; dark chocolate £4.34; fish £4.60; garlic £0.14. Regular, daily consumption of the Polymeal has been shown to reduce the risk of heart and artery disorders by 75 to 80 per cent – well worth the money.

## A Winner!
At Christmas 2004, the *British Medical Journal* ran a Polymeal competition based on six criteria: presentation, taste, texture, creativity, clarity of method, and adherence to the recommended types and quantities of the essential ingredients. The winner was general practitioner Dr Heather Hayward of Falkirk. This is her 3-course meal.

*Starter*:
## Roasted Red Pepper and Almond Dip, with lots of raw vegetables
80 g shelled almonds
285 g jar of roasted red peppers in olive oil
3 cloves of garlic, peeled and chopped finely
2 tsps of red wine vinegar
2 tbsps olive oil from the jar of peppers
salt and freshly ground black pepper

1      Preheat oven to 220°C (Regulo 7). Place almonds on a baking tray and roast for 8 minutes, until just golden. Allow to cool a little then whiz in a blender until fine.
2      Drain the peppers, reserving 2 tbsps oil.
3      Add peppers, garlic and vinegar to blender and whiz until coarse and with the machine running pour in the oil. Season.

Serve with carrot, cucumber, celery sticks and any available dipping vegetables.

*Main course:*
## Cod with Red Wine Sauce
4 x 275 g cod steaks
25 g butter
1 tbsp sunflower oil
seasoned flour
For the sauce:
25 g butter, diced and chilled
4 shallots, sliced
100 g streaky bacon, cut into strips
150 ml fruity red wine
159 ml chicken stock
2 tbsps chopped fresh parsley
seasoning

1   Season the cod steaks. Heat oven to 180°C (Regulo 4).
2   First put the 25 g of butter and oil in a roasting tin and melt over a medium heat. Lightly dust both sides of the cod steaks with the flour then lightly brown in the roasting tin. Remove and set aside.
3   For the sauce, gently fry shallots and bacon in remaining oil. Return the cod to the tin, cover with foil and roast for 15-20 minutes. Transfer fish to an ovenproof dish and keep warm.
4   Drain any excess fat from tin. Place over medium heat and add the wine to the shallots and bacon. Bring to the boil while stirring and scraping in the sediment. Add the stock and boil until reduced by two-thirds. Gradually add the chilled butter, swirling it in to thicken the sauce. Add parsley and season.
5   Pour a little sauce onto 4 warmed plates, place cod steaks on top and spoon remaining sauce over them.

Serve with boiled new potatoes, steamed broccoli and momentarily stir-fried mange-tout.

This recipe allows for three people to have a small glass of wine and one driver to enjoy the aroma in the fish!

*Finishers:*

## Marbled Chocolate Fondue

400 g plain bitter chocolate
100 g white chocolate
4 tbsps white rum or equivalent according to taste
500 g – 1 kg fresh fruit, for instance strawberries, cherries, bananas, pineapple, grapes, kiwis. . .
200 g nuts

1   Toast nuts in a dry pan or the oven until lightly browned. Cool then chop finely.
2   Prepare the fruit, cutting into bite-size chunks.
3   In two separate bowls over hot water or in the microwave melt the plain and white chocolate. Add 3 tbsps rum to the plain chocolate and 1tbsp to the white, if liked, or moisten with wine. Pour the plain chocolate into the fondue and lightly swirl in the white with a skewer. Keep just warm. Spear a piece of fruit and dip into the chocolate, then into the nuts – go on!

## Junk Food

This comprises empty calories, plus an excess of sweet, fatty and fattening food that requires nil or minimal preparation. It could be good for you if you were starving in Africa, when any calories would be a godsend, but otherwise it provides unhealthy, unbalanced nourishment. It often, but not necessarily, leads to overweight. Teenagers, men doing manual work, and middle-aged women at home alone for long periods, are the likeliest to stuff themselves with junk food – the lazy way of getting full but not fit.

## Age-related Diets

### Youth
Young people and men on their own:

- have a tendency to take too much alcohol, leading to drink/drive disasters;
- enjoy junk food snacks;
- have irregular, hurried and missed meals;
- generally eat processed, fried and sweet foods;
- consume fizzy drinks;
- have short periods of eating huge amounts – or nothing; and
- care liable to miss out on proteins, which are needed for building and repair work.

### Adults
For adults from 20 to 65, see General Dietary Requirements, page 7.

For the actively sportive, nutrition plays an important part in their wellbeing. There are no magic foods or supplements that enhance performance, but athletes in training require up to 8,000 kcal compared with the norm of 2,500 kcal a day. All women need proportionately more iron than men, and sportswomen need even more extra iron and calcium.

### The Elderly
The Third Age is marked by a reduced intake of food with mild weight loss, loss of height (bone) and muscle – but an increase in body fat. From the point of view of calories, less food is needed but the same range and variety of nutrients (carbohydrates etc.). There should be a reduction in fat, especially the saturated type like butter, and also of salt, but plenty of wholegrain cereal, fruit and vegetables. Sugar and alcohol need to be limited because of the smaller size of the liver.

For people in their Fourth Age (80-plus), with dentures and a weaker digestion, soft foods are often easier to manage and the dietary rules and restrictions that apply to the rest of us can be ignored. It is more important that the elderly enjoy their food and eat enough.

There are a number of foods that may trigger sensitivity or allergies:

- cow's milk and all dairy products;
- hen's eggs;
- fish, especially shellfish;
- some fruits, for instance strawberries;
- some vegetables, for instance cucumber;
- some nuts, especially peanuts;
- Chinese restaurant meals;
- additives, for instance preservatives, natural and artificial colouring, thickeners, flavour enhancers, sweeteners and antioxidants: these come under the control of the European Commission, with obligatory labelling; and
- wheat gluten, also barley and rye.

## Gluten-free Diet
Fresh milk, meat, fish, eggs, fruit and vegetables are all safe foods for the wheat-intolerant, but many processed foods do contain wheat. Fortunately gluten-free bread, biscuits, pasta and even communion wafers are available from healthfood shops and some supermarkets. It is important to keep strictly to the diet.

## Migraine reaction
Chocolate, cheese, red wine, citrus fruits and some fatty foods such as sausages can bring on a 'hot dog headache', a severe one-sided headache with nausea.

Where a sensitivity reaction or allergy occurs the culprit must be omitted from the diet, but not everyone reacts similarly. Some specific illnesses such as diabetes and kidney disease require a special diet as an integral part of their treatment.

## Elimination Diets
Sometimes it is not clear which is the food that is causing the trouble, so a process of elimination is the best way to detect it. The first step is to keep a comprehensive diary of what you have eaten and any reactions, and the second step is to omit all the foods on the suspect list for 2 to 3 weeks. After that, all being well, you gradually re-introduce these, one at a time, every 3 to 7 days. Finally, you are left with 1 or 2 items you must always avoid or, if you are lucky, none. Meanwhile, the foods least likely to upset you are:

- lamb, among the meats
- rice, of the cereals (polished)
- peeled, cooked potatoes and lettuce among the vegetables
- peeled pears among the fruits.

The oils of sunflower seeds and safflower are the mildest, and the drink least likely to cause a reaction is sugar and water. After one week on the restricted diet you should take a multivitamin pill daily.

## The Asian Soya and Spices Diet

Most Asian diets rely on soya, other vegetables, spices and herbs. They are stimulating to the bowel, and diverticular disorders are uncommon. Asian diets are only fattening if eaten to excess. They are rich in phyto-oestrogens, hormones derived from plants, and often ease women through the menopause without the need for hormone replacement therapy.

## The High Fibre Diet

Although fibre is either not absorbed at all or only partially digested, it is the most important ingredient that will ward off or reverse diverticular disorders. Fibre comes in two types: soluble or viscous, and insoluble. The former is the most important because of its valuable properties. First, it reduces dangerous fat levels in the blood, cholesterol, which tend to clog up the arteries causing high blood pressure and extra strain on the heart. Second, another life-saving effect of soluble fibre is the prevention of bowel cancer, the most common cancer in Britain, often occurring in people with diverticular disease.

### Foods Providing the Most Fibre

Foods high in fibre are specifically those containing 4 g or more of fibre in a normal serving. These include:

- bran-type breakfast cereals, for instance the range recently introduced by Kelloggs and based on All-Bran
- porridge oats
- oatmeal
- legumes: baked beans, kidney beans, butter beans, split peas and lentils: 100 g / 4 oz per serving
- dried fruit, e.g. raisins, currants, apricots, dates – up to 6 pieces
- nuts: 50 g / 2 oz of peanuts, almonds, walnuts, hazelnuts or Brazil nuts.

Take 1 or 2 servings daily from the above list.

## Good Sources of Fibre

Food providing 2 g of fibre per serving are:

- Cereals with 2 g or more fibre per serving, e.g. Weetabix, Shredded Wheat, Rice Crispies.
- 2 slices or a roll of wholemeal, multigrain, rye or cracked wheat bread or toast.
- Fruits: 1 whole apple, banana, pear, or orange, half a grapefruit or 100 g/4 oz of small fruits: raspberries, blackberries, strawberries or red or blackcurrants.
- Vegetables: 75 g/3 oz of runner beans, broccoli, brussels sprouts, carrots, sweetcorn, peas, parsnips, spinach, cabbage, jacket potato, bulgur rice.

Have 6 servings daily from the good sources list.

Raise the fibre content of soups, salads and casseroles by adding chickpeas, beans, lentils and the edible skins of fruits and vegetables.

Can there be too much of a good thing – in this case fibre? *Yes* – too much fibre causes the contents of the bowel to pass through the system too quickly, without absorbing enough of the vitamins and minerals. It can also cause over-frequent motions – diarrhoea. Fybogel is a commercial laxative made from the fibre of ispaghula husk, providing extra bulk, and is used to treat constipation. Too much causes abdominal pain, bloating and 'wind'.

# Mediterranean Food

The marvellous Mediterranean diet has the reputation of being the healthiest in the world, having the fewest victims of the big killers, coronary heart disease and stroke. It is also among the most delicious, with a flavour of sunshine, relaxation and holiday. It is especially beneficial to those of us who live in the northern parts of Europe.

Back in the early 1950s a group of doctors in Finland were disturbed to find that the death rate for their compatriots of age 60 upwards far exceeded that of other Europeans. The deadliest diseases involved the heart and arteries, but the commonest cancer involved the colon, and was often preceded by diverticulitis. Studies showed that the underlying cause of these illnesses lay in diet. Except in Finland, where the whole nation reformed its eating habits, nothing much happened in other countries apart from one or two localized experiments, for instance at Framingham in the United States and Lyon in France, until very recently. The latter showed that those on a strict Mediterranean diet recovered faster after an illness.

Professor Antonia Trichopoulou of Athens University published a remarkable paper in the usually staid *British Medical Journal* of 30 April 2005, followed by a broadcast by Richard Hannaford from the equally serious BBC in early May of this same year. It reported a study involving nearly 100,000 men and women in nine different European countries: Denmark, Sweden, Germany, France, the Netherlands, Greece, Italy, Spain and the United Kingdom. Each one was scored according to how closely they followed a typical Mediterranean diet, measured against their death rate. Those whose diet was nearest to the Mediterranean ideal had substantially fewer deaths.

The characteristics of the Mediterranean diet comprise:

- Plenty of fruit, vegetables, legumes and unrefined cereals: for instance, brown rice. The fibre in these foods stimulates the colon by filling it up naturally, unlike the chemical effects of laxatives. Fibre, because it is not digested, is not in the least fattening – although it may cause bloating with gas.
- Moderate to large amounts of fish, especially fatty types such as salmon and sardines.
- Moderate intake of alcohol. It has long been known to be beneficial to

the digestive tract, including the colon, also the heart in the middle-aged, to take 2-3 glasses of wine daily.
- Small amounts of meat and saturated fats. Saturated fats come from dairy products and red meat, neither of which is abundant in Mediterranean countries. They are also present in convenience foods, cakes, pastries and confectionary, pre-packed foods and takeaways.
- Plenty of unsaturated fats, especially the monounsaturated type such as olive and rapeseed oils. These are excellent for roasting and grilling as well as with salads.
- Polyunsaturated fats, found in vegetable oils like sunflower, safflower, soya, corn and most spreads.

Unexpectedly, the over-fifties in Northern Europe are more likely to rate themselves as in very good or excellent health than those from the southern part of the continent. Around 50 per cent of Swedes and Danes see themselves as really fit, compared with a mere 20 per cent of Spaniards, Italians and French. France, Sweden and Switzerland spend generously on health and reap the reward of a long life expectancy, while the United Kingdom, Greece, Italy and Spain try to run economically. In the case of the United Kingdom, there is a comparatively low life expectancy, whilst the Spaniards and Italians don't spend much money but live long. This is put down to their Mediterranean-style food.

A healthy lifestyle covers more than diet alone. The four health rules promoted by the government of the United States comprise:

- Don't smoke.
- Keep a normal weight: a body mass index of 25 or less.
- *Eat plenty of fruit and vegetables – the kingpin of a Mediterranean diet.*
- Take regular exercise: at least 10 minutes three times a day.

The benefits of keeping to these rules are huge and would eliminate most of our chronic disorders, but only 3 per cent of American citizens bother. Their children are getting steadily fatter. In Britain, levels of childhood obesity have risen from 9.6 per cent in 1995 to 14.9 per cent in 2003. Those from the poorest households are the fattest, eating more junk food than the others. (*Archives of Internal Medicine 2005*; 165-854-7)


## Mediterranean Dishes

**Italy**
Go for the native fare:

- a wide variety of cheeses including mozzarella, ricotta, Parmesan and Bel Paese
- tomatoes – raw, cooked or pureed
- red, green and yellow peppers
- purple egg plants
- artichokes
- lemons – and juice
- olives – and oil
- 'fruits of the ocean' – an abundant variety of fish including sardines, mussels, tiger prawns, red mullet and monkfish.

Pasta, said to have been introduced to Europe by Marco Polo, is part of many, if not most, Italian dishes. The varieties include lasagne, gnocchi, tagliatelle, spaghetti and the little envelopes, ravioli, each one concealing a tasty treat. This may be chicken, beef, cream cheese, Gruyere, Bel Paese or spinach.

Wine, of course, completes every Italian meal, from spicy Orvieto to delicate Lachrima Christi. It is used freely in cooking as well as for drinking.

## Minestrone Soup
1 rasher of lean bacon, lightly grilled
50 g/ 2 oz macaroni
1 onion
1 l/ 1 ¾ pt chicken stock
1 large carrot
50 g/ 2 oz French beans
50 g/ 2 oz lettuce or cabbage
50 g/ 2 oz sweetcorn
1 clove garlic
Parmesan cheese to garnish

Peel and chop all the ingredients and cook together gently for $1\frac{1}{2}$ hours or microwave until the vegetables are soft. Serve sprinkled with grated Parmesan cheese – enjoy!

## Polenta
This is a favourite, made from a yellow maize flour.
175-240 g/ 6-8 oz polenta
1 pt water

Boil the polenta in the water until it is thick and smooth. Spread it on a cool plate, then cut into slices or fashion into dumplings. Sprinkle generously with Parmesan and serve very hot.

## Spain
The beauty and drama of the Spanish scenery is reflected in the range and variety of the food. The local ingredients include many of those found in Italy: garlic, olives, oranges and grapefruit, salad vegetables and peppers. Saffron, rice and sardines are more characteristic of Spanish dishes, which are also a little heavier than other Mediterranean food. They are equally stimulating for the colon and a preventative against diverticular disorders.

### Gazpacho
A cold, refreshing soup made with diced or liquidized vegetables.
1lb / 450g large ripe tomatoes
1 large onion
2 cloves garlic
1 green pepper
1 red pepper
½ cucumber
2 slices whole wheat bread
3 tbsp olive oil
3 tbsp wine vinegar
300ml / ½ pt tomato juice
300ml / ½ pt water
Salt and freshly ground black pepper
To serve: small croutons and ice cubes

Place the tomatoes in a bowl and pour boiling water over them. After a few minutes the skins will loosen and it will become easy to remove the skins. Skin the tomatoes, discard the seeds and juice, roughly chop the flesh. Peel the onion and garlic and chop finely. Remove the pith and seeds from the peppers and dice. Peel and dice the cucumber. Cut the crusts from the bread and dice. Put the prepared vegetables and bread into a large bowl. Add remaining ingredients and season. Cover the bowl with foil and chill thoroughly – overnight is best for a good tasty soup.

You can partly blend the soup if you wish, or blend all of it, in which case offer small bowls of chopped onions, tomatoes, peppers, cucumber and croutons as a garnish — serve the soup with ice cubes floating in it.

### Conchas de Pollo a la Andaluza
240 g / 8 oz cold cooked chicken breast
2 tomatoes
2 gherkins

2 – 3 radishes
1 egg, hard-boiled
lettuce and parsley
For the mayonnaise:
2 egg yolks
pinch of salt and pepper
150 ml/ ¼ pt olive oil
1 tbsp white wine vinegar or lemon juice

Chop the chicken, tomatoes, gherkins, radishes and egg and put into a serving bowl. To make the mayonnaise, mix together the egg yolks seasoning, adding the olive oil slowly, drop by drop to prevent curdling. Finally add the white wine vinegar or lemon juice. Pour over the chicken salad and mix well. Serve cold.

## Cocido (Pork Stew)
450 g/ 1lb can chickpeas, washed
1 kg/ 2lb 4 oz chicken thighs
450 g/ 1 lb ham hock
450 g/ 1 lb cubed pork loin or shoulder
500 ml/ 18 fl oz white wine
1 l/ 1¼ pt water
1 l/ 1¼ pt chicken stock
6 spicy chorizo sausages
1 onion, sliced
4 potatoes, cubed
3 carrots, chopped
1 red hot chilli pepper, chopped
garlic mayonnaise and crusty bread to serve

Put the chickpeas, chicken, ham, pork, wine, water and stock into a large pan. Bring to the boil and simmer for 2 hours. Add the chorizo sausages, onion, potatoes, carrots and chilli. Cook for 45 minutes more. Just before serving, shred the meat off, the bone of the ham hock and add to the mixture. Serve with the garlic mayonnaise and thick chunks of crusty bread. Serves 6.

This is a traditional Spanish dish, typified by the chorizo and chilli pepper flavours.

## Greece

Greek civilization, including food and its preparation, has influenced the whole of the known world since Byzantine times. Like other Mediterranean countries, Greece is rich in vegetables such as aubergines, artichokes, asparagus, peppers, tomatoes and ladies' fingers, also fruits including lemons, limes, melons, figs and, of course, olives. Wine from local vineyards is plentiful, with sweet Samos particularly popular. Herbs and spices are used generously, with dill a favourite since time immemorial.

## Moussaka
2 aubergines, sliced unpeeled
2 onions, finely chopped
225 g / 8 oz minced beef or lamb
1 bay leaf
1 egg
250 ml / $\frac{1}{2}$ pt meat stock
150 ml / $\frac{1}{4}$ pt milk
150 ml / $\frac{1}{4}$ pt olive oil
sprinkle of salt and pepper
parsley to garnish

Fry the aubergines and onion, brown the minced beef or lamb, add the other ingredients then cook gently for 1 hour at 180°C/350°F/gas mark 4. Serve garnished with parsley.

## Greek Smoked Mackerel Salad
250 g / 9 oz ready-to-eat smoked mackerel fillets, skinned and cubed
100 g / $3\frac{1}{2}$ oz feta cheese, cubed in oil with herbs
8 cherry plum tomatoes, halved
$\frac{1}{2}$ cucumber, diced
12 black olives, pitted
juice of 1 lime or lemon
baby salad leaves and crusty wholemeal or pitta bread to serve

Place the smoked mackerel in a large bowl. Add the feta cheese, tomatoes, cucumber and olives. Mix together and serve on a bed of baby salad leaves. Drizzle the lime juice over the top. Accompany with crusty wholemeal or pitta bread. Serve as a starter or snack for 4, or as a main course for 2.

## Turkey

The Turkish diet dates back more than a thousand years. They invented the idea of cooking meat on a skewer – the kebab – and are credited with introducing rice from Persia to Europe. These are used in pilaffs. Spices and herbs, nuts and currants, make their dishes seem like a treat, especially sweets such as the famous Turkish Delight and fragrant rose petal jam. Fish dishes are a favourite – from the great variety of fish round the shores.

## Pilaff
225 g/ 8 oz rice
1½ pt meat stock
125 g/ 5 oz low-fat spread
1 tsp black pepper
pinch of salt
1 tbsp pine kernels
1 tbsp currants

Place all the ingredients into a large pan and cook gently for 1 hour or until the liquid is absorbed.

## Istanbul Eggs
olive oil
outside skins of 2 large onions
Turkish coffee
eggs according to number of people

Take as many eggs as required, break into a pan and cover with equal quantities of olive oil and Turkish coffee, and add the brown onion skins. Cover the pan and simmer very gently for ½ hour. The egg whites will be coffee-coloured and the yolks a brilliant saffron yellow. The eggs will taste like chestnuts.

All Mediterranean food is served with large quantities of locally-grown fruit and vegetables and accompanied by local wines. The recipes given here would all be completed with a handful of fruit and vegetables, preferably raw.

## France

### Toulouse Sausage Cassoulet
500 g/ 1lb 2 oz boned belly pork
500 g/ 1lb 2 oz shoulder lamb
250 g/ 9 oz piece of smoked bacon
450 g/ 1 lb Toulouse sausage (or any good sausage if not available)
2 onions
3 pink garlic cloves, peeled and chopped

splash of olive oil
35 g / 1¼ oz tomato purée
400 g / 15 oz can cannellini beans
2 bay leaves
1 l / 1¾ pt beef stock
freshly ground black pepper and pinch of salt
sprig of fresh thyme
handful of fresh parsley, chopped

Brown the pork, lamb and bacon on all sides. Cover and cook gently for 10 minutes. Cut the sausage into 3 cm/ 1¼ -inch pieces. Add the sausage, onions and garlic and a little oil. Stir. Now add the tomato purée, beans, bay leaves and stock. Season and cover. Cook for 2 hours on a low heat. Add the herbs and stir through. Serve with crusty French bread. Serves 4.

**Boeuf Bourguignonne**
900 g/ 2 lb topside of beef
freshly ground black pepper, very little salt
1 onion, sliced
fresh thyme
fresh parsley
1 bay leaf
olive oil
500 ml/ 18 fl oz red burgundy
100 g/ 3½ oz streaky bacon
15 g/ ½ oz flour
250 ml/ 9 fl oz beef stock
1 garlic clove, peeled and chopped
250 g/ 9 oz button mushrooms
butter for frying
rice or crusty bread to serve

Cut the beef into 2-inch cubes and put into a large bowl. Season. Add the onion, herbs, a little olive oil and the red wine. Marinate for 3 hours. Fry the bacon until soft; remove and set aside. Strain the marinade and reserve. Add the meat to the same pan and brown all over. Sprinkle the flour over to absorb the fat. Add the strained marinade, stir well and add the stock. Put in the garlic. Cover and simmer for 2 hours. Fry the mushrooms in butter, add to the meat and cook for another 30 minutes. Serve with rice or crusty bread. Serves 4.

This is a well-loved traditional dish full of the flavour of France – beef steeped in burgundy with garlic.

### Tuscan Slow-cooked Sausage and Pasta
1 tbsp olive oil
8 lightly-spiced Italian sausages
1 onion, finely chopped
2 garlic cloves, peeled and crushed
1 bay leaf
2 x 400 g/ 15 oz cans chopped tomatoes
nutmeg
freshly-ground black pepper and salt to taste
125 ml/ 4 fl oz natural yoghurt (the Tuscans use double cream, but this is too much saturated fat)
125 g/ 4½ oz Parmesan cheese, grated
300 g/ 10½ oz fresh penne pasta, cooked

Heat the oil in a pan. Skin the sausages and break them up; put into the pan and cook slowly for about 4 minutes. When they begin to brown add the onion, garlic and bay leaf. Cook gently for 30 minutes, when the onion should be soft and golden. Add the tomatoes and simmer for about 45 minutes until it becomes the consistency of a thick sauce. Finally add the nutmeg, seasoning, yoghurt and Parmesan. Remove the bay leaf. Serve on top of the cooked pasta. Serves 3-4.

Children in particular enjoy this, and adults appreciate a glass of Chianti with it.

### Frutti di Bosco Cup
300 g/ 10½ oz Galbani Santa Lucia Finetta Ricotta
100 g/ 3½ oz sugar
50 g/ 2 oz bitter chocolate
100 g/ 3½ oz mixed berries

Press the ricotta through a fine sieve, mix in the sugar (use less if possible) and the grated chocolate. Serve well chilled and decorated with berries. Serves 4.

### Marrow Provecal
1 medium-sized marrow, peeled
25 g/ 1 oz butter
1 medium onion, grated
1 garlic clove, crushed
1 green pepper, seeded and chopped

225 g/ 8 oz tomatoes
100 g/ 4 oz hard cheese, grated

Cut the marrow into 2.5 cm/ 1-inch rings and remove the seeds from the centres. Cut the rings into 2.5 cm/ 1-inch cubes. Melt the butter in a large pan and fry the marrow until golden (6-7 minutes). Transfer to a plate. Put the onion, garlic and green pepper in the remaining butter in the pan. Fry until pale gold. Add the tomatoes and marrow and mix well.

Place half the mixture in an ovenproof dish. Cover with 50 g/ 2 oz cheese, then the remaining marrow mixture. Sprinkle with the remaining cheese. Bake at 190°C/375°F/ gas mark 5 for 15 minutes.

## Italian Vegetable Soup
1 small carrot
1 baby leek
1 celery stick
50 g/ 2 oz green cabbage
900 ml/ 2½ pt vegetable stock
1 bay leaf
115 g/ 4 oz cooked cannellini beans
25 g/ 1 oz soup pasta, such as tiny shells, bows or stars
salt and freshly ground black pepper to taste
chopped fresh chives to garnish

Cut the carrot, leek and celery into 4 cm/ 2-inch long julienne strips. Finely shred the cabbage. Put the stock and bay leaf into a large saucepan and bring to the boil. Add the carrot, leek and celery, cover and simmer for 6 minutes until the vegetables are slightly softened but not tender. Add the cabbage, beans and pasta, then simmer, uncovered, for a further 4-5 minutes or until the vegetables are tender and the pasta is al dente. Remove the bay leaf and season to taste. To serve, ladle the soup into 4 warmed bowls and garnish with the chopped chives.

Use homemade vegetable stock rather than stock cubes to make a really delicious clear soup – fit for a special occasion.

## Tuscan Bean Soup
45 ml/ 3 tbsp extra-virgin olive oil
1 onion, roughly chopped
2 leeks, roughly chopped
1 large potato, diced
2 garlic cloves, finely chopped
1.2 l/ 2 pt vegetable stock

400 g/ 14 oz can cannellini beans, drained: reserve the liquid
175 g/ 6 oz Savoy cabbage, shredded
45 ml/ 3 tbsp fresh flat-leaf parsley, chopped
30 ml/ 2 tbsp fresh oregano, chopped
salt and freshly ground black pepper
75 g/ 3 oz Parmesan cheese, shaved
For the garlic toasts:
30-45 ml/ 2-3 tbsp extra virgin olive oil
6 thick slices country bread
1 garlic clove, peeled and bruised

Heat the oil in a large pan and gently cook the onion, leek, potato and garlic for 4-5 minutes, until beginning to soften. Pour on the stock and liquid from the beans. Cover and simmer for 15 minutes. Stir in the cabbage, beans and half the herbs, season and cook for a further 10 minutes. Spoon about one-third of the soup into a food processor or blender and process until fairly smooth. Return to the soup in the pan, adjust the seasoning and heat through for 5 minutes. To make the garlic toasts, drizzle a little oil over the slices of bread, then rub both sides of each slice with the garlic. Toast until browned on both sides. Ladle the soup into 4 bowls. Sprinkle with the remaining herbs and the Parmesan shavings. Add a drizzle of olive oil and serve with hot garlic toasts.

Mediterranean dishes are known as the healthiest as well as being so delicious – with an air of sun and holiday. The high fibre content and plentiful vitamins and antioxidants make them ideal for those at risk of diverticular problems.

# Snacks and Light Meals

The big risk of light meals and snacks is that only too easily they turn out to be quick and easy convenience or junk foods, packed with fat and sugar, and short on fruit and vegetables and the fibre they contain that is so valuable in the battle against diverticular disorders.

## Recipes

### Fruit and Nut Squares
115 g / 4 oz unsalted butter or spread, with a little extra for greasing
2 tbsp clear honey
1 egg, beaten
85 g / 3 oz ground almonds
115 g / 4 oz dried apricots, finely chopped
55 g / 2 oz dried cherries
55 g / 2 oz hazelnuts, toasted and chopped
25 g / 1 oz sesame seeds
85 g / 3 oz jumbo porridge oats

Grease a shallow baking tin. Beat the remaining butter with the honey until creamy, then beat in the egg and the almonds. Mix in the remaining ingredients and press the mixture firmly into the tin. Bake until golden brown and firm to the touch, about 20-25 minutes. Remove from the oven and leave for 10 minutes before marking into squares. Leave until cold before removing from the tin. Keep in an airtight container.

The oats release their sugar very slowly, making for a low GI value, and their fat content creates bodily warmth. A delicious snack whenever you like.

### Home-made Hummus
400 g / 14 oz can chickpeas, drained
2 tbsp tahini paste
4-6 tbsp virgin olive oil
4-6 tbsp lemon juice
2 crushed garlic cloves
1-2 tbsp hot water
pepper and a pinch of salt

red and yellow peppers cut into strips, celery and cucumber sticks to serve

Except for the crudités, put all the ingredients into a liquidizer with hot water and seasoning, making a dipping consistency. Refrigerate until wanted, then use as a dip with the crudités.

The raw garlic has antibacterial properties and a reputation for benefiting the heart.

## Stuffed Vegetables
2 tbsp vegetable stock
1 small onion, chopped
2 garlic cloves, crushed
2 tbsp tomato purée
6 ripe tomatoes, skinned and chopped
4 tbsp brown rice, cooked
25 g / 1 oz pine nuts, lightly toasted
1 tbsp fresh parsley, chopped
1 tbsp fresh mint, chopped
1 tbsp fresh basil, chopped
$\frac{1}{4}$ tsp ground cinnamon
juice of 1 lemon
black pepper

If stuffing aubergines or courgettes, halve them lengthways and hollow out each half with a teaspoon. Chop the scooped out flesh. Steam the empty shells over boiling water for about 4 minutes, then hold under the cold tap briefly and dry with kitchen paper.

If stuffing peppers, slice off the tops (save) and scoop out and discard the seeds.

If stuffing tomatoes, slice off the tops (save), scoop out seeds and flesh and add the latter to the rice mixture.

Heat the stock in a frying pan, add the onions and garlic and sauté, stirring, until translucent. Stir in the tomato purée, tomatoes, flesh of the chopped aubergines, or tomatoes or courgettes, cooked rice, pine nuts, herbs and cinnamon. Continue cooking for a couple of minutes. Stir in the lemon juice and season with pepper. Stuff the vegetables with the rice mixture and put the lids back on the peppers or tomatoes. Place on a lightly greased baking dish and bake for about 20 minutes.

This is a basic recipe for a balanced mixture to go with almost any vegetable.

## Spinach, Bacon and Herb Pie
butter or vegetable spread for greasing

225 g/ 8 oz shortcrust pastry
8 rashers back bacon, roughly chopped
3 medium onions, finely chopped
100 g/ 4 oz fresh spinach, finely chopped
3 tbsp fresh herbs of choice, chopped
3 eggs, beaten
100 ml/ 4 fl oz milk (plus a little to brush pastry top)
pepper and salt to taste
Optional extras: watercress, mushrooms, courgettes

Butter an ovenproof flan dish. Roll out the pastry and use half to line the dish. Lightly fry the bacon and spread over the pastry. Sauté the onions in a little butter until soft and mix together with the spinach and herbs (and any optional extras). Spread the mixture over the bacon. Whisk the eggs and milk together, season, and pour over the spinach mixture. Use the rest of the pastry to cover the mixture. Seal the edges and make a small hole in the lid. Glaze with a little milk. Cook for 30 minutes, until pastry is golden. Serve in slices.

### Herb-breaded Chicken
$1\frac{1}{2}$ slices wholemeal bread
$\frac{1}{4}$ tsp dried basil
$\frac{1}{4}$ tsp thyme
$\frac{1}{4}$ tsp oregano
$\frac{1}{4}$ tsp tarragon
$\frac{1}{4}$ tsp paprika
freshly ground pepper
4 chicken breasts, skinless and boneless

Pre-heat the oven to 180°C/350°F/gas mark 4. Make the bread into crumbs in a blender. Add the herbs and pepper to mix. Rinse the chicken under the cold tap, then shake off the water. Put the crumb mixture into a plastic bag with the chicken and shake until the crumbs coat the chicken pieces. Place the chicken in a single layer in an ovenproof dish. Bake for 18-20 minutes or until thoroughly cooked. Serve with raw or grilled halved tomatoes, or any left-over vegetables, hot or cold. Serves 4.

### Meatballs and Coriander Dip
40 g/ $1\frac{1}{2}$ oz raisins
200 g/ 8 oz lean minced lamb
75 g/ 3 oz water chestnuts, finely chopped
30 ml/ 2 tbsp spring onions, finely chopped

1 clove of garlic, finely chopped
½ tsp ground allspice
½ tsp cinnamon
freshly ground pepper
For the dip:
230 g/ 9 oz low-fat natural yoghurt
3 tbsp fresh coriander leaves, finely chopped
pepper to taste

Soak the raisins in hot water for 15 minutes, drain and chop. Combine the raisins, lamb, water chestnuts, spring onions, garlic, allspice, cinnamon and pepper to taste. Mix thoroughly. Shape into 25 bite-size balls. Arrange in a single layer in an ungreased baking dish. Bake uncovered in a pre-heated oven at 180°C/350°F/gas mark 4 for 15-20 minutes. To make the dip, in a small bowl combine the yoghurt, coriander and pepper to taste. Cover and refrigerate for 30 minutes.

Serve the hot meatballs with coctail sticks for dipping them into the sauce.

## Pitta Pizzas
4 wholemeal pitta bread rounds, 1520 cm/ 6-8 in
300 g/ 12 oz fresh mushrooms, thickly sliced
300 g/ 12 oz low-fat cottage cheese
50 g/ 2 oz grated low-fat cheddar or mozzarella cheese
5 ml/ 1 tsp dried thyme
5ml/ 1 tsp dried oregano
75 g/ 3 oz tomato purée
125 ml/ 4 fl oz water
5 ml/ 1 tsp granulated sugar
15 g/ ½ oz fresh chives or parsley, chopped

Cut round the edge of each pitta and separate into 2 rounds. Crisp on a baking sheet in a moderately hot oven (1-2 minutes). Simmer the mushrooms, covered, for 5 minutes or until tender, drain and set aside. In a bowl or blender combine the cottage cheese, mozzarella, thyme and oregano. Set aside. Combine the tomato puŕe, sugar and water. Mix well and spread over the pitta rounds. Top with the cheese mixture and spoon the mushrooms over the top. Bake in a pre-heated oven at 200°C/400°F/gas mark 6 for 10-15 minutes. Sprinkle with chives or parsley and serve. Serves 4.

Instead of mushrooms you can add a topping of red, yellow and/or green peppers, sliced onion, sliced tomatoes, sliced artichokes, chopped fresh basil and broccoli.

Instead of pittas you can substitute bread rolls, split in half or courgettes halved lengthways.

This recipe provides a useful supply of vitamin A, thiamine, riboflavin, calcium, fibre and iron and is an excellent supply of vitamin C and niacin. It is low in calories at just 286 kcals in a meal for four.

## Macaroni with Tomato and Tuna

1 tbsp olive oil
1 small onion, chopped
1 clove of garlic, crushed
398 g/ 14 oz can chopped tomatoes
125 ml/ 4 fl oz stock (any)
1 tsp dried or 2 tbsp chopped fresh basil
½ tsp dried or 2 tsp fresh rosemary
198 g/ 7 oz can tuna, drained
freshly ground pepper
15g/ ½ oz fresh parsley, chopped (optional)
225 g/ 8 oz macaroni

Heat the oil and cook the onion and garlic until tender. Add the tomatoes and break up using the back of a spoon. Stir in the stock, basil and rosemary and simmer, uncovered, for 10 minutes. Stir in the tuna and simmer for another 5 minutes. Season with pepper to taste and add the parsley. Meanwhile cook macaroni in boiling water until firm but tender, al dente. Toss with the tomato mixture and serve immediately.

This dish provides plenty of fibre and iron and is an excellent supply of vitamin C and niacin.

## Gratin of Winter Vegetables

2 tbsp vegetable oil
350 g/ 12 oz yellow turnip, cut into thin strips
125 ml/ 4 fl oz water
1 red pepper, cut into thin strips
100 g/ 4 oz onion, thinly sliced
300 g/ 10 oz courgettes, thinly sliced
75 g/ 3 oz mushrooms, sliced
4 medium tomatoes, cut in chunks
2 ml/ ½ tsp dried oregano
freshly ground pepper and pinch of salt
150 g/ 6 oz low-fat mozzarella cheese, grated
1 tbsp Parmesan cheese, grated

Heat the oil in a large pan. Add the turnip and cook until tender, about 10 minutes. Top up with water as necessary and add the red pepper and onions. Cook and stir for 2 minutes. Add the courgettes and mushrooms and cook, stirring, for 3 minutes. Add the tomatoes and turn the heat up high. Stir occasionally over 5-10 minutes. Add the oregano. Season with pepper and a little salt. Spoon the vegetable mixture into an ovenproof dish and sprinkle evenly with mozzarella and Parmesan cheese. Grill until the cheese has melted and slightly browned. Serves 8.

This satisfying, meat-free meal is low in calories and fat, but provides fibre, vitamin A, niacin and calcium and is an excellent supply of vitamin C despite the cooking. It can be refrigerated and reheated later for convenience.

### Salmon Spread with Capers
213 g/ 7½ oz can of salmon
25 g/ 1 oz capers, drained
25 g/ 1 oz celery, finely chopped
2 tbsp low-fat natural yoghurt
1 tsp lemon juice
hot pepper sauce
2 tbsp fresh parsley, chopped

In a small bowl flake the salmon, making sure the bones are well-crushed. Add the capers, celery, yoghurt and lemon juice and mix thoroughly. Add the hot pepper sauce to taste. Spoon into a serving dish and sprinkle with parsley. Serve as a spread with crackers or pitta bread or use to stuff vegetables such as cherry tomatoes or mange-tout.

Spring onions, chives, sweet peppers or fresh dill can be used instead of celery. Sock-eye salmon has the best flavour and red colour.

Preparation time can be measured in seconds. This tasty meal is very low in calories but is an excellent source of calcium and omega-3 fatty acids – good for bones and heart respectively.

### Spiced Lamb and Apricot Kebab
500 g/ 1 lb 2 oz lamb leg steaks, cut into 2.5 cm/ 1-inch pieces
125 g/ 4 oz ready-to-eat dried apricots
1 tbsp fresh mint, finely chopped
black pepper and pinch of salt
1 lemon, cut into 8 wedges
For the marinade:
1 clove of garlic, crushed
2 tbsp low-fat natural yoghurt

1 tbsp olive oil
1 tsp ground cumin
1 tsp ground coriander
1 tsp paprika
pinch of cayenne pepper
juice of 1 lemon

Make the marinade by mixing the garlic, yoghurt, oil, cumin, coriander, paprika, cayenne and lemon juice in a non-metallic bowl. Add the lamb, cover and refrigerate for an hour. Stir the apricots and mint into the lamb and season. Thread the lamb and apricots onto 8 metal or wooden skewers, placing a lemon wedge at the end. Discard the marinade. Preheat the grill at high and put the kebabs under it, on a baking sheet. Cook for 8-10 minutes, turning occasionally, until the meat is browned. Spoon the juices over the kebabs.

This is a nourishing dish, good for barbecues, served with raw vegetables or a salad.

## Chocolate Courgette Cake

115 g/ 3½ oz butter
2 eggs
300 g/ 10 oz sugar
1 tsp vanilla extract
125 ml/ 3 fl oz vegetable oil
4 tbsp cocoa
350 g/ 12 oz flour
1 tsp bicarbonate of soda
½ tsp ground cloves
½ tsp cinnamon
125 ml/ 4½ fl oz soured milk (just add 1 tsp of vinegar or lemon juice to milk)
200 g/ 6 oz semi-sweet baking chocolate, roughly chopped
2 small courgettes, grated

Preheat the oven to 180°C/350°F/gas mark 4 and grease a large baking tin. Cream the butter and eggs together. When they are creamy, gradually add the sugar, vanilla extract and oil. Blend or sift the dry ingredients together in a separate bowl and gradually add to the butter mixture. Then slowly blend in the soured milk. Add the chocolate pieces and grated courgettes. Bake for 40-50 minutes or until skewer inserted into the cake comes out clean. Eat hot from the oven or let it cool first. It is moist and tastes rather like carrot cake – delicious! Serves 6-8.

## Spicy Broccoli Pasta

400 g / 12 oz pasta
splash of olive oil
2 cloves of garlic, minced
1 chilli pepper, minced (optional)
400 g / ¾ lb sausages, sliced (optional)
2 heads of broccoli (or 1 if using meat)
salt and freshly ground pepper to taste
1 handful of fresh basil, torn into bits

Cook the pasta, and while it is cooking heat a large pan over a medium heat and add the olive oil, garlic and chilli. Add the sausage if required and sauté for about 5 minutes or until it is fully cooked. Then add the broccoli and sauté for another few minutes, until it is bright green and slightly tender but still crunchy. Add salt and freshly ground pepper to taste. Spoon over the pasta and sprinkle with plenty of basil. Serves 4.

## Sandwiches

These are a life-saver in an emergency, using whatever you have – eggs, ham, cheese, salad or other raw vegetables – with sliced bread, French bread or rolls, either Scandinavian open-style, or closed. They are useful for packed lunches for work or school, or on picnics or long journeys. They remain fresh better in the fridge and if the butter or spread comes right to the edges of the bread. Include something crisp, like lettuce, if the filling is soft, such as cottage cheese. Be generous with all fillings except mayonnaise.

### Toppings

1    Sliced egg and tomato, with mayonnaise and chopped chives.
2    Cottage cheese garnished with fresh fruit.
3    Sliced Double Gloucester cheese with black grapes and slices of apple.
4    Peeled prawns and mayonnaise garnished with paprika and lemon slices.
5    Sliced cooked sausage and coleslaw, garnished with parsley.
6    Cooked salmon and mayonnaise with sliced cucumber and lemon.
7    Bean salad and grated carrot with cherry tomatoes.
8    Sliced Cambridge blue cheese with grapes.
9    Cooked, sliced chicken with mayonnaise, chopped tomato and asparagus tips.
10   Grated Red Leicester cheese, cottage cheese and mustard and cress.

mixed nuts, dry roasted, unsalted 125 g/ 1 oz: 17 g fat, 197 calories
mixed nuts, oil roast, salted 125 g/ 1 oz: 19 g fat, 210 calories
potato chips (10): 7 g fat, 105 calories
pretzels, bread stick (5): trace fat, 59 calories
doughnut, yeast type: 11 g fat, 174 calories
chocolate-chip cookies (2): 6 g fat, 103 calories
milk chocolate bar (30 g): 10 g fat, 156 calories
ice-cream (125 g/ 5 oz): 8 g fat, 142 calories
fruit yoghurt (1 pot, 150 g): 2 g fat, 142 calories
fruit ice-lolly: 0 fat, 50 calories
apple: 0 fat, 84 calories
banana: 0 fat, 105 calories
1 Club biscuit (22 g): 6 g fat, 114 calories
Digestive biscuits (2): 5 g fat, 118 calories
RichTea biscuits (2): 2 g fat, 59 calories
Fig rolls (2): 2 g fat, 144 calories
1 currant bun, (60 g) : 5 g fat, 181 calories
1 wholemeal scone with no butter or spread (60 g): 9 g fat, 196 calories

Mini-snacks may be taken between meals, if you are still unsatisfied after a meal or if you have low energy for no particular reason. You should drink or have a light bite every 1½–2 hours  little and often. Choose one item only from the above list.

# Weights and Measures

## Weights

| | |
|---|---|
| 1 ounce (oz) | 30 g |
| 2 lb 3 oz | 1 kg |

## Liquid or Volume Measures

| | |
|---|---|
| British Imperial pint (pt) | 20 fl oz |
| American pint | 16 fl oz |
| 1¾ English pints | 1 litre |
| 1 tsp | 5 ml |
| 1 tbsp | 15 ml |
| 1 English teacup | ¼ pt (1 gill) |
| 1 English breakfast cup | ½ pt |
| English | American |
| 1 lb butter or spread | 2 cups |
| 1 lb flour | 4 cups |
| 1 lb granulated or castor sugar | 2 cups |
| 1 lb treacle or syrup | 1 cup |
| 1 oz flour | 1 heaped tbsp |
| 1 oz treacle | 1 level tbsp |
| 1 oz jam | 1 level tbsp |
| ½ oz butter | 1 tbsp smoothed off |

## Portions of Fruit and Vegetables

Large fruits: 1 apple, 1 orange, 1 banana
Medium-sized fruits: 2 plums, 2 satsumas, 2 kiwi fruits
Small and soft fruits: 1 cupful of raspberries, strawberries, blackberries, blackcurrants, grapes
Dried fruit (raisins, etc.): 15 ml / 1 tbsp
Fruit juice: 150 ml / ¼ pt
salad: 1 desert bowl
vegetables, raw, cooked or frozen: 30 ml / 2 tbsps